In
Balance
for Life

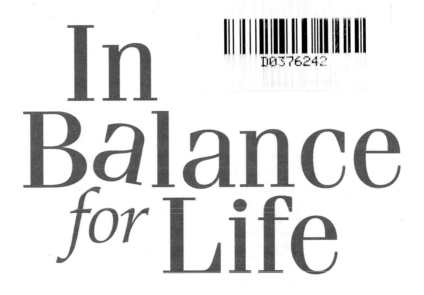

Alex Guerrero

SQUAREONE
PUBLISHERS
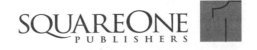

COVER DESIGNER: Phaedra Mastrocola
EDITOR: Joanne Abrams
TYPESETTER: Gary A. Rosenberg

The information and advice contained in this book are based upon the research and the personal and professional experiences of the author. They are not intended as a substitute for consulting with a health care professional. The publisher and author are not responsible for any adverse effects or consequences resulting from the use of any of the suggestions, preparations, or procedures discussed in this book. All matters pertaining to your physical health should be supervised by a health care professional. It is a sign of wisdom, not cowardice, to seek a second or third opinion.

Square One Publishers
115 Herricks Road
Garden City Park, NY 11040
(516) 535-2010 • (877) 900-BOOK
www.squareonepublishers.com

Library of Congress Cataloging-in-Publication Data
Guerrero, Alex.
    In balance for life : understanding and maxmimizng your
body's Ph factor / Alex Guerrero.
        p. cm.
    Includes bibliographical references and index.
    ISBN 0-7570-0264-1 (pbk.)
    1. Acid-base equilibrium—Health aspects. 2. Acid-base imbalances—Prevention.
I. Title.
QP90.7.G84   2005
616.3'992—dc22
                                                                    2004027289

3448 4302
10/06

Printed in the United States of America

10   9   8   7   6   5   4   3   2   1

Contents

Acknowledgments, v

Introduction, 1

1. "Houston, We Have a Problem," 5

2. Essentials for Good Health, 17

3. The pH Factor, 39

4. Many Diseases—One Primary Cause, 59

5. Getting Back in Balance, 77

6. Supplementation—The Extra Edge, 103

7. The 14-Day Diet and Sample Recipes, 125

Conclusion, 161

Glossary of Terms, 163

Bibliography, 173

Index, 175

Acknowledgments

There are so many people who deserve credit for this book that it's hard to know where to start. So I'll go back to the beginning and thank my late father-in-law, whose valiant fight with cancer began me on my journey. Thanks, Vay, for your love, your encouragement, and your advice. I miss you.

Thanks, too, to all of my professors at SAMRA University for imparting their knowledge and guiding me along my path. And to all of my clients for their constant support (and sometimes nagging) to get me to write. I would be remiss if I did not thank my personal assistant/protector/girl Friday, Debbie, for everything—your support and friendship have been invaluable to me. Thanks, as well, to David Knight, my agent. God put you into my life to finally get the ball rolling and help me get my jumbled thoughts onto paper. Thanks also to Larry Trivieri, Jr., whose talent is enormous, and whose research helped make this book all that it is. And, of course, my heartfelt gratitude to my publisher, Rudy Shur, who believed in this project from the start, and who guided it to its completion with wisdom and skillful insight.

My biggest thank-you goes to my lovely wife, Alicia. Words cannot express the joy of these last seventeen years of marriage. Thanks for never doubting me and always being my anchor and support, and thanks for our beautiful children—Liz, Josh, Bree, Justin, and Katie—my true motivators.

My final debt of gratitude goes to my Creator, without whom I am nothing. My deepest prayer is for truth to prevail.

Introduction

Today, it is practically impossible to go anywhere without hearing about how our country is facing a health crisis of major proportions—the prices of drugs are skyrocketing; millions of citizens go without health insurance; and a third of our population already suffers from some form of degenerative disease. While our politicians, economists, and health experts argue about how best to face this problem, few, if any, seem to have any realistic long-term solution.

There is, however, an answer. It is a solution that isn't complicated, doesn't require billions of tax dollars, and doesn't need a giant bureaucratic overseer. The answer is . . . good health. If fewer people needed pills to lower blood pressure, decrease cholesterol levels, or stimulate their love lives, think about the impact it would have on our health-care system. If fewer people suffered from the severe pain of arthritis, rheumatism, and other degenerative diseases, think how much emptier doctors' offices would be. And if the incidence of cancer started to drop sharply, consider how much less sorrow and grief there would be in our lives.

The sad truth is that health is something the majority of people in this country are lacking. The incidence of chronic illness is at an all-time high. Just as alarming, even among people who don't have any obvious symptoms of disease, lack of energy seems to be epidemic. Certainly, it is the number-one complaint among my clients, as well as the clients of my colleagues. Yet, paradoxically, at no time in history has such a wealth of health information been available to us, as evidenced by the abundant supply of books, newsletters, magazines, seminars, and websites all devoted to providing health information. So why are we so unhealthy as a nation? And, more importantly, what can be done about it?

That's what this book is all about. I wrote it to answer these questions, and to empower you with all the information you need to reclaim and maintain your health and vitality, now and for the rest of your life. After years of careful research, study, and observation, I can say with absolute confidence that the solution to this country's health problems does exist and that it can be summarized in one word—Balance!

Our bodies are designed to be healthy. This is a scientific fact. Regardless of your current state of health, if you follow my easy-to-use system for restoring and maintaining the balance your body requires for optimal health, I guarantee that you will experience a noticeable difference in how you feel. This is a bold claim, to be sure, but I make it with confidence, because each day, I witness how clients suffering from every conceivable malady experience dramatic improvements in their health after implementing the very principles you will discover in this book. Even if you are already healthy, these principles can help you, just as they have helped the world-class and professional athletes who consult me every day.

In the pages that follow, you will learn not only how your body works, but also how you can begin to move it from a state of degeneration and fatigue to a state of regeneration and vitality. You will also learn about the number-one key for doing so—proper acid-alkaline balance, also known as the pH Factor.

The information I will be sharing with you is not new. In fact, the principles that support it have been scientifically verified time and time again by researchers throughout the world. For the most part, however, they remain all but ignored by conventional and alternative health-care providers alike. As a result, our society is increasingly burdened with health-care problems.

Fortunately, the principles presented in this book are easy to understand, and even easier to implement. By applying them to your daily life, you will be taking back control of your health and starting down the road to optimal vitality. No matter what health challenge you may presently be facing, you can increase your well-being by adopting the guidelines that follow. This is my message to you: You don't have to be sick!

In the chapters that follow, you will learn:

❏ The full extent of our nation's health-care crisis, and the primary factors that contribute to it.

❏ The absolute essentials for achieving excellent health, and the means by which you can easily ensure that they become part of your daily life.

❏ The important role that the pH Factor plays in health and overall balance of the body; the reason that this role is misunderstood or ignored by most health-care practitioners; and the reason why unhealthy pH levels—a disruption of proper acid-alkaline balance—are at the root of all disease conditions.

❏ Why the foods you eat are the key to good health, and how you can take charge of your health by knowing what foods to eat, how you should prepare these foods, and exactly when these foods should be consumed.

❏ The nutritional supplement program that will take your health to the next level.

❏ My 14-Day Diet Plan to quick-start your journey to vibrant vitality.

If you are ready to reclaim your health, turn the page and read on.

1

"Houston, We Have a Problem"

ecently, the Associated Press ran a news item entitled *Study: We're Eating Ourselves to Death.* The gist of the story was that America's unhealthy eating habits are about to overtake smoking as the number-one preventable cause of death and illness. According to the same report, in 2000, poor diet, obesity, and physical inactivity accounted for approximately 400,000 deaths in this country—a full 16 percent of all recorded deaths that year.

Grim as these statistics are, they don't begin to tell the full story of our nation's health-care crisis. As Drs. Robert S. Ivker and Robert A. Anderson point out in their book *The Complete Self-Care Guide to Holistic Medicine*, "[T]he United States, the world's wealthiest nation, is entering the twenty-first century with its population beset with record levels of chronic illness." Conservatively, it is estimated that over 100 million Americans suffer from some type of chronic ailment, and that number continues to increase. Equally alarming is the epidemic of obesity in this country, something health officials have now identified as our number-one health problem. According to the National Institutes of Health, over $100 billion is spent each year on problems related to obesity.

Children and teenagers are at particular risk for turning obese. According to Drs. Ivker and Anderson, obesity among children and teenagers has steadily increased since 1970 (50 percent in children and 40 percent in teenagers). In addition, one out of every six children in America suffers from other health problems such as attention deficit hyperactivity disorder (ADHD), asthma, autism, dyslexia, and obesity. And in recent decades there has been a stark rise in "syndrome conditions," such as chronic fatigue syndrome, fibromyalgia, and environmental illness. Unlike specific disease conditions, these disorders mask themselves in a wide range of symptoms, making their diagnosis and treatment difficult to properly assess. Then, too, there are the less bothersome symptoms, such as foggy thinking, fatigue, and minor aches and pains that afflict so many of us from time to time. Although they don't count as disease per se, they nonetheless take their toll, affecting our well-being and our ability to be productive. All told, we as a nation are not very healthy. This is why we spend nearly $2 trillion a year on health-care costs—far more than any other country in the world, and a sum that experts predict will continue to rise. Clearly, something is very wrong with this picture. With so much money and so many resources annually being allocated to health care, why are we getting sicker instead of healthier?

Health experts answer that question by listing a variety of factors, and no doubt, you are aware of many of them. The most notable include:

❏ Unhealthy eating habits.

❏ Lack of exercise.

❏ Stress.

❏ Proliferation of environmental pollutants.

Let's briefly examine each of these factors in turn.

THE STANDARD AMERICAN DIET

The relationship between diet and health is no secret. In 1988, Surgeon General C. Everett Koop issued his "Surgeon General's Report on Health and Nutrition," in which he wrote, "One personal choice seems to influence long-term health prospects more than any other— what we eat." In the same report, Dr. Koop pointed out, "When [health] problems arise, they result from imbalances in nutrient intake and from harmful interaction with other factors." Yet, despite this clear warning, many Americans continue to subsist on a diet of "super-sized" processed foods that are high in calories and all but devoid of essential nutrients such as vitamins and minerals. Medical research has conclusively shown that foods containing saturated and hydrogenated fats, white flour and other refined carbohydrates, and chemical additives are major contributors to poor health and disease. The result is that we as a nation are eating ourselves to death and growing obese in the process.

Obesity

An estimated 34 percent of all American adults are obese, along with 25 percent of school-aged children. Yet, paradoxically, Americans spend over $110 million *each and every day* on diet and weight-loss programs. That's more than $40 billion a year, with little in the way of results to show for it. Research shows that 95 percent of all people who lose weight by dieting not only gain the weight back, but within three years, wind up weighing more than they did before their diets began. Further compounding the problem is the fact that overweight people have a higher risk of premature death, and are typically more prone to developing diseases such as arthritis, diabetes, cancer, cardiovascular illness, gastrointestinal disorders, gout, sleep disorders, respiratory problems, high blood pressure, hernias, and gall bladder disease. But weight gain is not the only aspect of our diet that is contributing to the current health-care crisis.

Food Quality

Even people who are not overweight—as well as people who avoid eating junk foods—are finding it increasingly difficult to stay healthy. The cause of this can be traced to the commercial farming methods used in the harvesting of our nation's food crops. These methods employ large amounts of chemical fertilizers that encourage rapid plant growth, but return little or none of the vital minerals removed from the soil by growing plants. As a result, since the mid-twentieth century, the mineral content of American soils has steadily declined, as has the nutritional value of the fruits and vegetables that are grown in such soil. This decline in mineral-rich soil has resulted in an increase in malnutrition, setting the stage for further disease.

Additionally, commercially grown fruits and vegetables are usually laced with pesticides, and by time they reach the marketplace, may also contain preservatives and other synthetic additives. Similar problems exist in the commercial meat, poultry, and dairy industries. The products produced by these industries are derived from animals that are given unhealthy injections of growth hormones, as well as antibiotics used to counteract the unsanitary conditions in which the animals live. Antibiotics, along with food dyes, are also used in the harvesting of "farm-raised" fish. Once the animals are slaughtered, the foods are then irradiated, ostensibly as a safety precaution. This practice is now common despite objections from health safety advocates who claim that irradiation can pose additional health risks. Research has also shown that irradiation further depletes the nutritional value of foods.

Genetically Altered Food

A recent development impacting the American diet was the introduction of genetically engineered foods within the commercial farming industry. Dubbed "Frankenfoods" by health experts critical of their use, GMO (genetically modified organism) food crops have had their genetic codes combined with the genes of unrelated plant species. Although proponents of this practice claim that it improves the foods' nutritional value and taste, a survey conducted by the Union of Concerned Scientists found that 93 percent of the time that genetic engineering is employed, its goal is to make food production and processing easier and more profitable—not to improve the nutrient content of the foods. This year, a more recent study by the Union of Concerned Scientists found that more than two-thirds of conventional food crops have been polluted with genetically modified material due to the drift of inserted genes into adjoining, non-GMO food crops.

"Diet Monotony"

Yet another contributor to our poor health is the lack of variety in our diets. "Diet monotony" is a term I use to describe the fact that most of us tend to eat the same foods day in and day out, thus severely limiting our nutrient intake. In addition, our typical food choices are based on what tastes good, not on what foods are good for us. By and large, the standard American diet consists of a steady stream of wheat and dairy products, meat, and poultry, with inadequate amounts of fresh fruits and vegetables, seeds and nuts, and other fiber- and nutrient-rich foods. Over time, "diet monotony" not only results in nutritional deficiencies, but also can lead to the development of food allergies and sensitivities.

Water

Chronic dehydration is another important aspect of poor diet. The world's leading expert on this problem, Dr. F. Batmanghelidj, MD, author of *Your Body's Many Cries for Water,* has researched this subject exclusively for over three decades. According to his findings, the vast majority of Americans unknowingly suffer from chronic dehydration. Simply put, they lack the water needed to carry out virtually every vital function of the human body. Water comprises between 70 to 75 percent of the human body, and 85 percent of the human brain. Next to oxygen, nothing is more essential to life than water. Without it, we would die within a few days.

Most people wait for the sensation of thirst before drinking a glass of water, but according to Dr. Batmanghelidj's research, dehydration occurs in the body long before we begin to feel thirsty. That's because we are losing water all the time. For instance, water exits our bodies each time we exhale. The mere act of breathing eliminates as much as two cups of water every day. We lose another two cups of water each day through perspiration, and more than two additional pints through urination. Under normal circumstances, therefore, we lose the equivalent of eight to ten cups of water a day, which is why it is so important to continually drink adequate amounts of water.

THE HEALTH RISKS OF A SEDENTARY LIFESTYLE

We Americans are becoming increasingly sedentary to the detriment of our overall health. Numerous studies attest to the importance of regular exercise to good health, and show that habitual lack of exercise is a primary contributing factor to poor health and premature death. In a study of nearly 8,000 men and women, it was found that those who did not exercise increased their risk of premature death by an astonishing 400 percent, compared with those who exercised regularly. Some researchers consider lack of exercise to be a greater risk factor for decreased life expectancy than the combined risks posed by cigarette smoking, obesity, hypertension, and high cholesterol. As Drs. Ivker and Anderson point out, "Simply put, being unfit means being unhealthy."

Among the conditions caused or aggravated by lack of exercise and regular physical activity are anxiety; depression; poor sleep; reduced mental function and acuity; diminished aerobic capacity and increased oxygen deprivation in the bloodstream; increased risk of heart disease, cancer, and other diseases; reduced muscle strength and flexibility; impaired metabolic rate; impaired digestion and increased risk of gastrointestinal disorders; diminished self-esteem and overall feelings of well-being; lack of energy; chronic fatigue; increased weight gain and overall percentage of body fat; diminished experience of positive attitudes and emotions; increased body tension; and increased likelihood of hormonal imbalances. Conversely, research shows that all of these conditions tend to improve when an exercise program that combines aerobics, stretching, and strength conditioning becomes part of a regular health regimen.

Despite the overwhelming evidence linking exercise to good health, lack of exercise is perhaps even more common than poor diet. Too many of us are "trapped" in our daily routines. We have busy schedules, obligations, and jobs that require us to sit at our desks for hours on end. And then we spend our evenings unwinding on the couch watching TV. If this describes your own daily routine, you need to consider making exercise a part of your life. Information on safely and easily doing so is presented in Chapter 2.

STRESS—THE MALADY OF OUR MODERN WORLD

Stress is seemingly inescapable in today's fast-paced world. According to the Centers for Disease Control and Prevention (CDC), it is also a primary contributing factor to 85 percent of all disease conditions. In 1998, researcher Bruce Lipton, PhD, a cellular biologist at Stanford University, set the figure even higher. In a published scientific paper, Dr. Lipton stated that unresolved, internalized stress plays a major role in 95 percent of all illness.

Although certain types of stress are a normal part of life, when stress is prolonged and unresolved, serious health issues can arise. It is therefore vital to learn to recognize the signs of stress as a means of preventing its health-sapping effects. Common indications of stress include heart palpitations, constricted throat or breathing, headaches, sweaty palms, stomach "butterflies," weariness or exhaustion, pain, nausea, ulcers, and diarrhea.

While not a disease, per se, stress can aggravate already existing health conditions. This can set the stage for a vicious circle, whereby stressful feelings worsen the disease, which in turn creates further stress, thus preventing the body from healing. High levels of stress have been shown to increase susceptibility to disease, suppress immune function, and contribute to hormonal imbalances. For the most part, stress falls into four categories: physical, psychological, psychosocial, and psychospiritual.

Causes of physical stress include physical trauma, such as infection or injury; either too much or too little physical activity; environmental pollution; illness caused by viral, bacterial, or fungal agents; fatigue; lack of oxygen; low blood sugar (hypoglycemia); nutritional and/or hormonal imbalances; food allergies or sensitivities; dehydration; musculoskeletal imbalances; and dental problems.

Common sources of psychological stress include unresolved emotions such as fear, resentment, sadness, anger, and grief. They also include unhealthy attitudes caused by information overload, excessive worry, self-criticism, a driven sense of perfection, and a sense of "losing control" of one's life.

Psychosocial stress can be caused by relationship difficulties, social isolation, and a lack of social support. Psychospiritual stress is commonly the result of a crisis of faith or values, questions about one's purpose in life, a lack of meaningful work, or an involvement in day-to-day activities that do not reflect one's core beliefs.

Regardless of the type and source of stress you may experience, on a biochemical level, your response to it will usually be the same. Hans Selye, MD, one of the most important stress researchers in the history of mind/body medicine, determined that our biochemical response to stress follows a consistent pattern that he termed the *General Adaptation Syndrome.*

When stress occurs, it primarily affects your body's autonomic nervous system (ANS), which is often likened to your body's autopilot. The ANS is responsible for regulating your breathing, digestion, heart rate, and other physiological activities, without your having to consciously be aware of them. There are two aspects of the ANS—the *sympathetic nervous system*, which governs how your body's energy is expended, and the *parasympathetic nervous system*, which conserves your body's energy supply.

During the General Adaptation Syndrome process, the body's sympathetic nervous system is flooded with hormones secreted by the endocrine glands, and constricts the body's involuntary muscles and blood supply. Simultaneously, the body's parasympathetic nervous system is also stimulated, seeking to bring the body back into a state of relaxation. When stress becomes chronic, this two-fold action can be likened to having your feet on the gas and brake pedals at the same time. Before long, this "stop-go" action wears your body down, exhausting your energy supplies and setting the stage for illness.

A TOXIC BREW—OUR POLLUTED PLANET

Since the 1940s, beginning with the pioneering research of the late Theron Randolph, MD, holistic health-care practitioners have been aware of the relationship between the health of our bodies and the health of our environment. Since that time, they have warned us that environmental toxins and pollutants play a direct role in the creation and persistence of a wide range of disease conditions, including allergies, arthritis, cancer, cardiovascular disease, chronic childhood illnesses, endocrine disorders, gastrointestinal conditions, skin disease, musculoskeletal disorders, respiratory illnesses, and nervous system disorders.

Despite this awareness of the link between environmental toxins and disease, the proliferation of these harmful agents for the most part continues unabated, as evidenced by the following statistics cited by health journalist Larry Trivieri, Jr., in his book *The American Holistic Medical Association Guide to Holistic Health:*

❑ An estimated 20,000 different types of pesticides are currently in use, with over 4 billion pounds used worldwide each year.

❑ Fifty percent of all pesticide use occurs in the United States.

❑ Worldwide, 25 million people succumb to pesticide poisoning each year.

❑ According to the Environmental Protection Agency (EPA), 98 pesticides and over 600 other chemicals have been detected in U.S. drinking water since 1984.

❑ According to the EPA, the average American spends 90 percent of each day indoors, breathing air that can be as much as 100 times more polluted than outdoor air.

❑ More than 400 toxic chemicals have been identified in human tissue.

❏ Currently, an estimated 80,000 chemicals are regularly in use, with an additional 1,000 to 2,000 more being added to this list each year.

❏ Only 3 percent of the chemicals in use have ever been tested to determine whether they are toxic or carcinogenic (cancer-causing).

❏ In 1998 alone, the United States released approximately 500 billion tons of toxic chemicals into the environment.

In addition to these startling facts, researchers have found that nearly 70 million Americans now live in locations that exceed safe smog standards, over 3,000 chemicals have been added to the United States food supply, and approximately 10,000 chemicals are used in commercial food processing and storage. Further adding to this problem is the widespread use of everyday products such as gasoline, paint, household cleansers, and dry cleaning fluids, not to mention the proliferation of antibiotics, growth hormones, and genetically modified food agents in our food supply, already discussed. Based on these facts, creating and maintaining a healthy home and work environment has become more important than ever. In Chapter 2, I will show you effective ways in which you can positively control or influence your personal environment.

THE BODY'S ACID-ALKALINE BALANCE

All of the factors discussed so far are obviously important, and must be addressed if health is to be achieved and maintained. Yet even when they are addressed, the health gains that are achieved will not be lasting if a much more basic goal remains overlooked: Bringing the body back into an acid-alkaline balance. Unfortunately, it is this most vital aspect of health that is so often ignored by health-care practitioners.

Yet the concept of acid-alkaline balance is not new. In 1933, for instance, William Howard Hay, MD, wrote a book entitled *A New Health Era*. In it, he wrote, "[W]e depart from health in just the proportion to which we have allowed our alkalis to be dissipated by introduction of acid-forming food in too great amount." Dr. Hay went on to write, "It may seem strange to say that all disease is the same thing, no matter what its myriad modes of expression, but it is verily so." In Chapter 4, we will explore this very same premise and you will discover that Dr. Hay was absolutely correct.

Arthur C. Guyton, MD, regarded as a world authority on human physiology, echoed Dr. Hay's views a few decades later when he wrote *The Textbook of Medical Physiology*, which remains essential reading for today's medical students. In it, Dr. Guyton says, "[T]he regulation of hydrogen ion concentration is one of the most important aspects of homeostasis." In plain English, "hydrogen ion concentration" means pH, or the acid-alkaline balance, and "homeostasis" refers to the body's inherent self-regulating mechanisms, which seek always to maintain equilibrium, or balance, within the body's systems.

When I talk about acid-alkaline balance, I am referring to the pH of your blood. There are other pH levels related to other parts of the body—the saliva, urine, and body tissues, for instance—but from my clinical experience, blood pH provides the best indication of your overall health. The blood pH reading reflects the concentration of hydrogen ions in the blood. In a state of optimal health, blood pH is 7.365 on a scale of 1 to 14. When blood pH moves lower than this level, the body shifts into an acidic state, and if pH rises above the healthy norm of 7.365, an overly alkaline state can occur. When either a state of acidity or over-alkalinity becomes chronic, the stage is set for disease to take hold. This is similar to what happens when body temperature falls or rises from the ideal norm of 98.6 degrees for a prolonged time. Most people with chronic health problems have a blood pH level that is chronically acidic (below 7.365), but disease may also be due to a chronically elevated (overly alkaline) pH level. What follows are some of the health hazards that can result when the acid-alkaline balance becomes disrupted.

Disruption of Cell Function

Every cell in your body requires a balanced pH in order to function properly. Over time, an acid-alkaline imbalance impairs cell function, forcing the body to compensate. This, in turn, disrupts the body's attempts to maintain homeostasis. When that happens, a state of *disease* takes over. The body's weakest organ systems are attacked first. These first sites will vary, depending on a person's genetic predisposition. With sustained imbalance, the process moves on to impair additional systems as they too become weakened.

Susceptibility to Pathogens

Contrary to popular belief, we do not become ill simply because we come in contact with germs or other pathogens. The truth of the matter is that all of us are exposed to potentially harmful bacteria, viruses, and fungi—collectively regarded as pathogens or germs—each and every day of our lives. Yet only some of us become sick, while the rest of us remain healthy. As you will see, it is the acid-alkaline balance that makes all the difference.

It is only when pH becomes imbalanced—usually in an overly acidic state—that bacteria, viruses, and fungi are able to thrive and multiply in the body. When pH is balanced, pathogens are easily identified and eliminated by the body's immune system.

Candidiasis

Candidiasis is the name given to a systemic infection of *Candida albicans,* a type of yeast that naturally occurs in your gastrointestinal (GI) tract. Under healthy conditions, when pH is balanced, the spread of *Candida* is kept in check, and its presence is beneficial to the body. *Candida* serves to assist in the various processes overseen by the gastrointestinal system; it helps to digest food, assimilate nutrients, and eliminate waste products. But when acid-alkaline imbalance occurs, *Candida* can easily overgrow its normal bounds, settling throughout the body and causing a wide range of health conditions, some of which can even be fatal. Candidiasis is a very common, yet often overlooked, chronic health condition in the United States today.

Other Health Problems

As you will discover in Chapters 3 and 4, chronic acid-alkaline imbalance can also result in a host of other health risks and disease conditions. These include weight gain, allergies, fatigue, mood swings, memory problems, neurological conditions, blood sugar imbalances, GI disorders, and respiratory conditions, to name just a few. Infants and children are also susceptible to the ravages of acid-alkaline imbalance. It can also play a role in rashes, ear infections, hyperactivity, learning disabilities, attention deficit disorder (ADD), and even poor self-esteem. The good news—proven to me every day by the clients I see—is that all of these conditions can be resolved once the proper steps are taken to correct pH imbalances. By following the correct course of action, my clients experience lasting improved health and greater overall vitality.

CONCLUSION

As we have seen, our nation is faced with a seemingly overwhelming health-care crisis, with an escalating number of people afflicted with chronic disease conditions. But hopeless as the situation may appear, I know that the system I am about to share with you can dramatically improve your health and the lives of your loved ones, just as it has improved the health of the thousands of men and women with whom I have worked.

Now that we've examined the factors that are at the core of our nation's health-care crisis, let's move on to explore and understand all of the primary elements that are essential for good health.

2

Essentials for Good Health

The human body is a truly miraculous creation. It is designed to continuously maintain its healthy functioning through the process of homeostasis, its system of self-regulating mechanisms. Unfortunately, in today's world of stress, environmental pollution, and adulterated foods, it is becoming increasingly difficult for our bodies to operate the way God and Nature intended. Due to all the stresses exerted on our bodies during the course of our day-to-day lives, homeostasis is difficult to maintain. Once our bodies fall out of balance, a state of dis-ease sets in, which, if left uncorrected, ultimately leads to illness of one sort or another.

The key to becoming and staying healthy, therefore, lies in doing all we can to ensure that balance is maintained. In this chapter, I will share with you the essential elements, both internal and external, that you can use to achieve a consistent state of disease-free vitality. But before I do so, let's take a moment to reflect on what being healthy truly means.

ARE YOU HEALTHY?

If you are reading this book without any obvious health complaints, most likely your answer to this question is "Yes." But is that really true? I meet people all the time who tell me they are healthy and free of symptoms. Yet when I examine them, it often turns out that this isn't the case at all. While they are correct in telling me they are not suffering from any obvious signs of illness, in point of fact, most of them admit to having some complaint. They express their frustration at having less energy or less flexibility than they would like. They tell me of minor yet nagging aches and pains, constant stress, or an inability to get a good night's sleep.

If these nagging symptoms sound all too familiar to you, you should know that such complaints are common to millions of people in our nation. And then there are the tens of millions more who suffer from far more serious health problems, as we discussed in Chapter 1. The fact is that we have forgotten what being truly healthy actually means. Health is not merely a condition of being symptom-free. It is a state of abundant energy and mental and emotional well-being.

On page 19, I present a simple test that will enable you to discover how healthy you really are. As you answer the questions, note how many attributes of health you are now experiencing or, conversely, how few of them you are enjoying. This test is by no means conclusive, but it does provide you with an easy way to assess your health in general terms. It can also help you determine the areas of your health on which you may need to work. Now that you've gained a better understanding of your current health status, let's examine the factors that are absolutely essential for good health.

Thomas Edison once wrote, "The doctor of the future will give no medicine, but will interest his patients in the care of the human frame, in diet, and in the cause and prevention of disease." This is precisely my aim in writing this book. I have the utmost admiration for the many marvelous achievements of our modern system of conventional medicine, which is unrivaled when it comes to dealing with acute medical emergencies. And I am in favor of the thoughtful use of pharmaceutical drugs. But my primary aim as a healer is to help you prevent disease from occurring in the first place. To do so, it is important that you take responsibility for your own health, and commit to taking the necessary steps to ensure it. These steps involve providing yourself with all that your body needs to be healthy. The seven essentials for optimum health are:

1. Proper diet and nutrition.

2. Adequate water intake.

3. Regular exercise.

4. Restful sleep and relaxation.

The "How Healthy Are You?" Quiz

For each point, fill in the most appropriate number from 1 to 5—1 indicating that you experience the described feeling or condition rarely; 3, that you experience it occasionally; 5, that you experience it often. Make sure to answer honestly.

1. You go through each day with abundant energy. _____

2. You fall asleep easily and sleep deeply. _____

3. You awaken each morning feeling well-rested and ready to tackle the day. _____

4. You are within 20 pounds of your healthy body weight. _____

5. You feel fit and limber. _____

6. You are physically strong. _____

7. You feel physically attractive. _____

8. You have a positive overall mental outlook and can cope with daily challenges. _____

9. You regularly experience joy and feelings of satisfaction. _____

10. You live and work in healthy environments that support your well-being. _____

11. You have strong and emotionally fulfilling bonds with your family and/or friends. _____

12. You feel connected to the world around you. _____

Total Points _____

First add up the number of points you have written. If your total points fall below 30, your level of health may be easily compromised. If it falls between 30 and 50 points, your health is better than that of most people, but is subject to fluctuation. If, however, you have scored above 50 points, you have managed to create a stable health environment for yourself.

5. Healthy home and work environment.

6. Stress management.

7. Healthy acid-alkaline balance in your body fluids and tissues.

The remainder of this chapter is devoted to providing you with a better understanding of each of the first six essentials for vibrant health. It also includes sound advice for meeting your basic health needs. Chapter 3 deals entirely with the seventh essential: acid-alkaline balance and the pH Factor.

DIET AND NUTRITION

A healthy diet is the cornerstone of optimal health. Maimonides, the famed twelfth-century physician, wrote, "No illness which can be treated by diet should be treated by any other means." This sentiment echoed that of Hippocrates, the Father of Western Medicine, who more than a thousand years earlier had said, "Let food be thy medicine, and medicine thy food." Such advice goes directly to the heart of this book—to its goal of creating and achieving a healthy acid-alkaline balance.

Why is diet so important to your health? Because the foods you eat supply the fuel your body needs to perform its thousands of daily functions. The better your fuel supply, the better able your body is to generate energy, repair itself, and resist invading pathogens. Conversely, eating poorly diminishes your body's ability to maintain optimum functioning.

Given the important relationship diet has to health, one would think that health experts would agree upon what a healthy diet actually is. Unfortunately, one of the public's leading complaints relates to the vast amount of conflicting nutritional advice provided by today's so-called health experts. This is due, in no small part, to the many books published each year touting the "latest and greatest" cure-all diet. Simply check the current list of nonfiction bestsellers for today's "breakthrough"—from low-fat to no-fat, from low-carb to high-protein. Considering how these books so often contradict one another, it is no wonder that so many people are literally "fed up" with dietary advice.

Eating healthy should not be an exercise in fads. And it does not have to be, as you will soon discover. The key to eating well is to eat foods that provide your body with what it needs to maintain a healthy pH. In Chapter 5, I will show you how to do so easily and without confusion. For now, let's list and examine the most significant guidelines for eating healthy.

Eat Fresh Fruits and Vegetables. Fresh fruits and vegetables should be a daily staple of your diet. They are rich in vital nutrients and enzymes, and high in fiber. Be sure to eat at least a portion of your daily vegetable intake raw, since high cooking temperatures can destroy their nutrient and enzyme contents. (More information on the merits of eating raw versus cooked vegetables is provided in Chapter 5.) Lightly steamed vegetables are another healthy alternative.

Eat a Variety of Foods. As we discussed in Chapter 1, many people today are deficient in essential nutrients because they routinely eat a limited amount of foods, meal after meal. Not only does such diet monotony limit nutrient intake, but it also can lead to food allergies and sensitivities, both of which are common health conditions. By eating a wide variety of foods, you will have a much better chance of avoiding such conditions, and will also increase your nutrient intake.

Eat Organic Foods. Whenever possible, I recommend that you eat organic foods. Organic fruits and vegetables have been shown to have a higher nutrient content than nonorganic produce, and are also free of harmful pesticides, preservatives, and other chemicals used to grow most commercial food crops. Similarly, your meat and poultry choices should ideally be free-range and free of the hormones and antibiotics commonly given to commercially raised animals.

Maximize Your Intake of Essential Fatty Acids. Contrary to popular belief, all of us require a certain amount of fat in our diet. Fats act as the body's energy reserves, and serve as a primary form of insulation, helping to maintain normal body temperature. In addition, fats assist in transporting oxygen, help in the absorption of fat-soluble vitamins, and act as natural anti-inflammatory agents. Fats also help nourish the skin, nerves, and mucous membranes. The best sources of dietary fat are essential fatty acids (EFAs), particularly omega-3 and omega-6 fats. Many people have an excess of omega-6 fats in their diet, compared with omega-3, so you'll want to be sure to get the proper balance. Good sources of omega-3 EFAs include sardines, wild game, flaxseed and flaxseed oil, walnuts, pumpkin seeds, and canola oil.

Eat Plenty of Fiber. The standard American diet supplies only 25 to 33 percent of the fiber necessary for optimum health. Yet research shows that a high-fiber diet is closely associated with a lower incidence of heart disease, high blood pressure, certain types of cancer (especially colon and rectal cancer), diabetes, constipation, hemorrhoids, gall bladder disease, and gastrointestinal conditions such as colitis and diverticulitis. Good sources of fiber include fruits, vegetables, bran, rolled oats, brown rice, and other complex carbohydrates.

Eliminate "Junk" and Fast Foods. Simply put, these foods are unhealthy and, when eaten on a regular basis, will inevitably lead to disease. Moreover, they are typically high in calories and low in nutrient content, and are among the leading causes of acid-alkaline imbalance. If you are truly committed to your health, you will avoid eating such foods altogether.

Eliminate Sugar. The average American consumes 150 pounds of sugar each and every year. This is the equivalent of more than 40 teaspoons of sugar a day, which goes a long way towards explaining why we are so unhealthy as a nation. Sugar's many harmful effects include an increased risk of heart disease, a weakened immune system with increased susceptibility to infection, excessive insulin production, an increased production of harmful triglycerides, diminished mental function, increased feelings of anxiety and depression, an increased risk of cancer, and systemic yeast overgrowth (candidiasis).

To fully eliminate sugar from your diet, it is necessary to read food labels, since sugar is a common ingredient in packaged foods in the forms of fructose, sucrose, corn syrup, lactose, and maltose. In general, foods that are frozen, canned, processed, or cured are likely to be high in sugar.

Eliminate Unhealthy Fats. As mentioned earlier, certain fats are essential for good health. Unfortunately, many of us, instead of eating foods rich in healthy fats, consume harmful trans-fatty acids and saturated fats, both of which have been linked to a host of disease conditions, including arteriosclerosis, heart attack, angina, cancer, kidney failure, and obesity. Trans-fatty acids are found in hydrogenated oils, which are used to make margarine, commercial cookies and crackers, commercial peanut butter, commercial cereals, and many other packaged foods. Saturated fats are found in red meat, milk, and milk products such as butter and cheese, as well as in palm oil, palm kernel oil, and coconut oil.

Minimize Caffeine. It is estimated that more than half of all Americans are addicted to caffeine, primarily through their daily intake of coffee. While caffeine in moderation—no more than 200 milligrams per day—is relatively harmless, too much regular caffeine consumption can contribute to a wide range of health problems and can decrease platelet stickiness, thus interfering with the blood clotting process. It can also cause a loss of calcium in the body, thereby disrupting the acid-alkaline balance.

Minimize Your Salt Intake. Salt is another ingredient that is far too prevalent in many people's diets. Although a certain amount of salt is required by the body to carry out its many functions, too much salt can cause problems. When salt intake is excessive, water is drawn into the bloodstream, increasing blood volume. This, in turn, can increase blood pressure levels, and can also interfere with the ability of the body's lymphatic system to eliminate waste matter from the cells.

Eliminate Refined Carbohydrates. Refined carbohydrates—found in white bread, pasta made from white flour, instant mashed potatoes, white rice, chips, sugar-laden commercial cereals, and many other processed foods—are an unfortunate staple of the standard American diet, and pose additional health risks. The most common negative effects of the regular consumption of refined carbs are excessive insulin production, excessive fat storage, and elevated blood sugar levels. Eventually, regular consumption can lead to serious health conditions such as obesity and diabetes.

Drink Alcohol Only in Moderation. Although in recent years a number of studies have indicated that a moderate consumption of wine or beer may provide health benefits, such as reduced stress and improved digestion, not everyone is able to drink alcohol only in moderation. In addition to the well-known social problems associated with alcohol abuse, excessive alcohol consumption has been directly linked with a variety of disease conditions, including hypertension, diabetes, obesity, gastrointestinal disorders, impaired liver function, candidiasis, cancer, impaired mental function, and behavioral and emotional problems. Moreover, although many people drink in order to feel better, research conducted by the National Cen-

Should Nutritional Supplements Be Part of Your Daily Health Routine?

In an ideal world, a healthy diet rich in a wide variety of organic foods would allow us to meet all of our nutritional needs each day. Unfortunately, we live in a world that is far from ideal. In addition to daily life stresses, our world is burdened with pollutants in the water, air, and soil. Even our nation's organically grown foods are harvested from soils that are greatly deficient in the trace minerals necessary for nutrient-rich fruits and vegetables.

Compounding the problem is that much of our nation's food supply does not reach us for weeks or months after it is harvested. Often, it is shipped, frozen, stored, and warehoused, losing nutrient value at every stop. Pesticides, insecticides, preservatives, additives, and other chemicals are also widely used in food production. For these reasons, nutritional supplementation can often be a valuable component of your daily health regimen. Supplementation alone, however, is by no means an acceptable substitute for a healthy diet. Moreover, there is no such thing as a "one size fits all" recommendation when it comes to the use of nutritional supplements. This is because of each person's unique *biochemical individuality*, a phrase coined by researcher Roger Williams, PhD, in the 1930s. Williams found that the amount of nutrients required for optimal health can vary by as much as 700 percent from person to person, due to genetic makeup as well as factors such as age, diet, environment, and stress levels.

Depending on a person's needs, I sometimes recommend a nutritional supplement program as a complement to my dietary program. If necessary, tests to determine your nutritional needs and imbalances may be advisable. These can be ordered by your physician, who ideally will be experienced in the use of nutritional medicine. As a preventive measure, supplementing with a multivitamin/mineral formula can be a good idea. There are many such formulas available at your local health food store. For better absorbability, choose one that is of food grade quality, as opposed to a supplement composed of synthetic vitamins and minerals. I will have more to share on this subject in Chapter 6.

ter for Health Statistics has found that alcohol consumption can result in pronounced feelings of loneliness and depression.

By following the above guidelines, you can significantly improve your health over time. The key is to commit yourself to making these practices a regular part of your daily life. The dietary recommendations that I will share with you in Chapter 5 will enable you to quickly and easily progress down the road to lasting health and vitality.

ADEQUATE WATER INTAKE

Approximately 70 percent of our bodies are made up of water—80 percent in infants—and water is the medium through which all of our body functions occur. Water is essential for:

❏ Healthy brain function and conduction of nerve impulses.

❏ Proper metabolism and digestion.

❏ Delivery of oxygen into the bloodstream.

❏ Proper kidney and urinary function.

❏ Proper regulation of body temperature via perspiration.

❏ Joint lubrication and muscle function.

❏ Healthy respiratory function.

❏ Proper function of the lymphatic system and the elimination of waste products via the urine.

When we fail to drink enough water each day, over time, many health problems can arise. These include:

❏ Reduced brain size, leading to impaired neuromuscular coordination and mental function.

❏ Constipation and diarrhea.

❏ Diminished oxygen supply in the bloodstream, resulting in inadequate delivery of oxygen and nutrients to all body organs and muscles.

❏ Excess body fat.

❏ Kidney stones and urinary tract infection.

❏ Poor muscle tone and muscle size.

❏ Diminished resistance to infection.

❏ Sinus congestion.

❏ Musculoskeletal pain and related health conditions.

❏ Edema (water retention).

❏ Impaired metabolism.

❏ Blood thickening, which can increase the risk of heart attack and hypertension.

❏ Buildup of toxins in body cells, tissues, and organs.

Based on the above, it is easy to see why water is so essential to our health. Yet, according to Dr. F. Batmanghelidj, the world's foremost authority on the relationship of water to health, most people are chronically dehydrated and aren't even aware of it. As explained in Chapter 1, under normal conditions, each of us eliminates two to two and a half quarts of water each day through exhalation, perspiration, and urination. Exercise and exposure to heat further increase water loss, especially in dry climates. That is why it is so important to replenish the water you lose by drinking water throughout the day.

Although you may not think you are dehydrated, there's a good chance that you are. In his book *Your Body's Many Cries for Water,* Dr. Batmanghelidj points out that the body's most recognizable thirst signal, "dry mouth," is "the *last* outward sign of extreme *dehydration.*" Other signs of dehydration include fatigue, respiratory problems, and the various symptoms listed above. The appearance of your urine is also an indication of your level of hydration. If your urine is cloudy and/or yellow, orange, or brown in color, it is more than likely you are not getting an adequate supply of water each day. When you are properly hydrated, your urine will tend to be light and nearly clear in color.

Drinking adequate water does not mean increasing your intake of coffee, soft drinks, commercial teas, milk, processed juices, or alcohol. Not only do these substances actually serve to further *increase* dehydration, but they can significantly impair your body's healthy acid-alkaline balance. Many health practitioners now recommend that you drink six to eight glasses of water a day, but Dr, Batmanghelidj recommends that you drink half an ounce of water for every pound of your weight. This means that a 150-pound person should drink about nine glasses of water a day. If you are a particularly active exerciser, you can increase this ratio to two-thirds of an ounce per pound of body weight. On the other hand, if you consume large amounts of fresh fruits and vegetables every day, your daily water intake can be slightly decreased, since these foods are 85 to 90 percent water by weight.

Be sure that the water you drink is pure and filtered—not chlorinated or fluoridated. Distilled water is also not recommended, since it is devoid of necessary minerals and can actually leach them from your body. Initially, as you increase your water intake, you may experience a more frequent need to urinate. This will not last for more than a few days, after which your body should adjust to the increased intake of fluids.

To get in the habit of drinking adequate water, drink it throughout the day. However, do not drink more than four eight-ounce glasses in any one-hour period. It is also best to drink one or two glasses of water upon arising, at least thirty minutes before breakfast. As a general rule, always drink water at least thirty minutes before or after a meal, as consuming a good deal of water during meals can interfere with digestion.

EXERCISE

Research has shown that, on average, people who make exercise a regular part of their lives live longer and enjoy better health than people who have sedentary lifestyles and don't exercise. But even though the benefits of exercise have been well-established by numerous scientific studies, we have become increasingly sedentary as a nation. This alarming trend is especially true of our children, 25 percent of whom are overweight or obese.

What follows are only a few of the many benefits afforded by regular exercise:

❑ Increased muscle strength and flexibility.

❑ Improved digestion.

❑ Increased energy.

❑ Improved quality of sleep.

❑ Improved mental function.

❏ Increased longevity.

❏ Improved cardiovascular function.

❏ Healthier muscle-to-fat ratio.

❏ Healthier self-image and greater self-esteem.

❏ More frequent experiences of joy and positive attitude.

❏ Improved aerobic capacity.

❏ Decreased tension and stress.

❏ Fewer incidences of anxiety and depression.

❏ Greater resistance to infection.

❏ Reduced risk of cancer and other chronic/degenerative diseases.

The best exercise programs include a mix of activities that increase aerobic capacity, muscle strength, and flexibility. Aerobic exercises help to increase the supply of oxygen to your muscles, which in turn creates more energy. (The word *aerobic* literally means *with oxygen.*) The most common and convenient forms of aerobic exercise include brisk walking, jogging, swimming, bicycling, hiking, and rebounding (jumping on a mini-trampoline). Treadmills, rowing machines, stair climbers, and stationary bikes can also provide an excellent aerobic workout. The key to long-term success is finding an activity that you enjoy, and committing to it on a regular basis. If possible, exercise outdoors, as the combination of fresh air and bright sunshine will make your activities more enjoyable and provide even greater health benefits.

Building and maintaining muscle strength is also essential for good health. This can be accomplished through the regular practice of exercises such as push-ups, chin-ups, and sit-ups, or through a weight-training program that uses free weights or weight machines. If you are new to such exercises, it is a good idea to seek your physician's approval before beginning. Once you get the okay to begin, consult with an exercise specialist or personal trainer, who can help you design an aerobic and weight-training program that will most closely suit your goals and needs.

There are a variety of ways to achieve and maintain flexibility, beginning with basic stretching exercises. Yoga, Pilates, and Tai Chi are other popular forms of exercise that promote greater flexibility and improved muscle strength. Flexibility is important for a number of reasons. It promotes greater muscle strength and function; it better enables muscles to perform efficiently, with less risk of strain and injury; it enhances circulation; it increases the health of your body's connective tissue, tendons, and ligaments; and it improves posture.

The Importance of a Healthy Spine to Overall Health

Even though musculoskeletal problems such as backache are among the most common complaints, spine health is one of the most overlooked aspects of overall health. Not only does a properly aligned spine minimize the risk of musculoskeletal disorders, but it also ensures optimal function of the nervous system, which regulates all of the body's systems through the network of nerves that extend from the twenty-four vertebrae of the spine to every organ and gland of the body.

When your spine becomes misaligned—a condition known as *subluxation*—the nerve impulses transmitted by the brain become impaired. This results in diminished function on the part of the body systems to which the brain sends its messages. The primary structural cause of nerve interference is pressure placed on the nerves by misaligned vertebrae. Chronic muscle tension, muscle spasm, and constricted connective tissue within the musculature can also contribute to this problem by pulling and keeping the vertebrae out of alignment. Once the spine is restored to its proper alignment, nerve function improves, resulting in improvements in the rest of the body's systems, as well.

A regular program of stretching or other exercises designed to promote flexibility is an excellent means of maintaining proper spinal function. If you already suffer from spinal misalignment, a number of health-care treatments can help you address the problem. The most popular of these are chiropractic, bodywork and massage, and osteopathic manipulation. Other therapies such as yoga, Tai Chi, Rolfing, the Alexander Technique, and Bowen Therapy can also be most helpful. Being aware of and addressing spine and muscle tension can lead to dramatic long-term improvements in your overall health.

SLEEP AND RELAXATION

Restful sleep and regular periods of relaxation are two other essential elements of good health. Lack of sleep can lead to diminished immune function, and can negatively affect both mood and mental alertness. Prolonged periods of nonrelaxation can cause stress to build up, creating chronic tension in your musculature. Yet poor sleep affects tens of millions of Americans each year, while an even greater number complain of how "stressed out" they are due to lifestyles that aren't conducive to relaxation.

Although sleep is a succession of five recurring stages, for our purposes, we will break it into two basic categories—heavy sleep and light sleep—that you should ideally cycle through each night. During heavy sleep, your body's self-repair and healing mechanisms are revitalized. During the REM (rapid eye movement) stage of light sleep, dreams help the body release stored stress and tension. Insomnia (the inability to fall asleep) and inadequate sleep are the two most common sleep-related problems that interfere with these processes of revitalization and tension relief. Fortunately, both of these problems can usually be resolved. By making the following simple changes in your daily routine, you will be well on your way to getting a good night's sleep.

Make Dietary Adjustments. It is well known that eating too late in the evening can result in poor sleep. For that reason, it is a good idea to refrain from eating for three to four hours before retiring. If a good night's sleep remains elusive, you'll want to consider other dietary factors as well. Caffeine, salt, sugar, and alcohol consumption can all interfere with your ability to get a good night's sleep. Just as important, a diet that is not conducive to maintaining your body's acid-alkaline balance can be a major culprit. By following the dietary recommendations mentioned earlier in this chapter and in Chapter 5, you should be able to avoid the dietary pitfalls that can prevent you from enjoying adequate sleep.

Drink Herbal Teas. Herbal teas have been used for centuries to promote restful sleep. Among the most popular and safe herbal tea remedies for sleep problems are chamomile, hops, and valerian root. Chamomile is particularly useful if your inability to sleep is related to muscle tension or gastrointestinal upsets, since it has been scientifically shown to ease both problems. Hops tea is useful if you suffer from nervous tension or sleep disturbances. And in Germany, valerian root has been approved as an over-the-counter remedy for general sleep disorders. For best results, drink the tea forty-five minutes before retiring.

Get Adequate Exercise. According to sleep researchers, many people who suffer from insomnia also lead sedentary lifestyles, which can add to their sleeping problems. Adopting a light to moderate exercise routine is often all that is necessary to improve sleeping patterns. Consider a leisurely walk of one or two miles in the early evening. Remember, however, that an evening exercise routine can be counterproductive if the exercise is vigorous, as this can cause sleeplessness due to overstimulation.

Use Breathing Exercises. Because of their calming effect, breathing exercises can greatly enhance your ability to fall asleep. Each of the following two exercises requires only a few minutes to perform, and when practiced regularly, can become a highly effective trigger for the sleep response. Choose the breathing technique that suits you best.

To perform the first exercise, lie on your back with your eyes closed and the lights out. Begin gently but deeply inhaling, taking as much air into your lungs as is comfortable. At the end of the first two exhalations, exhale fully, drawing in your abdomen. At the end of the third exhalation, hold your breath for as long as you can. Repeat the process two or three times, or until you feel sleepy.

To perform the second exercise, breathe in for a count of four; then hold your breath for another count of four. Exhale fully. Then again hold your breath for a count of four. Repeat the entire process until you feel sleepy. Three or four repetitions are usually adequate.

Gain Relief From Stress. Sleeping problems are often related to stored stress and tension. Fortunately, relaxation techniques can help you manage stress, and thereby enhance both your ability to sleep and your overall health. See the discussion on page 34 to learn more about relaxation techniques.

Create an Optimal Sleep Environment. The environment in which you sleep in is an often-overlooked factor that can contribute to a restless night. Be sure that your bedroom is kept clean and free of dust, that the room receives adequate fresh air, and that your mattress is not uncomfortable. Also be aware that you may be sensitive to the materials in your pillow, blankets, and sheets. As a general rule, cotton sheets and blankets and feather pillows are better than items made from synthetic materials.

If you have a television set in your bedroom, either move it into another room or unplug it. Your bedroom should be maintained as your sleeping quarters, not as an entertainment center. By watching TV or reading in bed, you will create an environment that keeps your conscious brain active. But by training yourself to believe that your den is for watching television or reading and your bedroom is for sleeping, you will increase your odds of falling asleep. Also make sure that the temperature in your bedroom is kept at a comfortable level. Temperatures that are too hot or cold can significantly interfere with sleep.

Finally, if you have an electric clock, be sure that it sits as least eight feet away from your bed. To further avoid electromagnetic pollution, try not to sleep near cell phones and stereos, television sets, or computer equipment unless they are unplugged. Finally, if you still find yourself unable to fall asleep, get out of bed and out of the bedroom. Sit or lie down comfortably in another area of the house, and engage in a quiet, relaxing activity, such as reading or listening to music. When you find yourself becoming drowsy, return to your bedroom and go to bed.

HEALTHY HOME AND WORK ENVIRONMENTS

As we've discussed, the environment in which we live is increasingly becoming burdened with toxic chemicals and other pollutants. The range of health conditions associated with these toxins is large and continues to grow, which is why it is very important that you do all you can to ensure that you live and work in a toxin- and pollutant-free environment. In particular, you need to do your best to breathe clean air, drink pure water, and minimize your exposure to substances in the environment that can cause disease. As a further precaution— especially if you live in an area of poor air quality, such as a major city—consider the use of antioxidant vitamin supplements, such as vitamins A, C, E, and beta-carotene, all of which can help protect against the free-radical damage caused by environmental pollutants.

Improve the Air Around You. To ensure the quality of the indoor air you breathe, consider placing plants throughout your home and at work. Plants create moisture and add more oxygen to indoor environments. They also filter out carbon monoxide and organic chemicals.

You might also consider using a negative ion generator, which can significantly improve indoor air quality. Negative ions are air molecules that contain an abundance of electrons. The benefit of using a negative ion generator is similar to that of breathing fresh ocean air, which also has a high concentration of negative ions. You will feel energized and more alive. Studies also indicate that the use of a negative ion generator can enhance respiratory function, filter out indoor air pollutants, and safeguard against the proliferation of harmful molds and bacteria.

If the air you breathe in your home or work environment is dry, you might also benefit from the use of a humidifier. Dry air, especially when it is cold, can be a major factor in chronic respiratory conditions such as bronchitis and sinusitis, and can also contribute to allergies, according to Dr. Robert Ivker, author of *Sinus Survival*. Dr. Ivker recommends that your indoor air have a relative humidity of 35 to 55 percent—a condition that can easily be achieved with the use of a room humidifier. He strongly advises the use of warm-mist humidifiers, but cautions that you must clean them at least once a week. Unlike other humidifiers, they require no filter and can be operated using regular tap water.

Use People- and Pet-Friendly Materials. Synthetic materials that emit potentially toxic substances—such as particle board, fiberboard, and plastics—can also diminish indoor air quality. Formaldehyde found in insulation materials and plywood can pose problems, as well. Commercial cleaning products are yet another potential source of indoor pollution, as they often contain toxic chemicals.

Fortunately, for each synthetic or toxic material or product, there are natural alternatives. Throughout your home and work environments, be sure to use products made of wood, cotton, metal, and other natural materials. When choosing cleaning products, select from among the many nontoxic alternatives that are now widely available.

STRESS MANAGEMENT

With stress playing a role in as much as 95 percent of all disease conditions, the importance of proper stress management cannot be overemphasized. For just as stress contributes to illness, managing and reducing stress at home and at work can help promote healing. All of us are exposed to stress triggers, or *stressors,* each and every day. In my experience, I have found that the stressors themselves aren't as important as the way in which you cope with them. Fortunately, you can significantly improve your ability to successfully deal with stressful stimuli and events. Health-care professionals offer numerous helpful approaches, including biofeedback therapy, hypnotherapy, guided imagery training, and psychological counseling. But there are also a number of steps you can take on your own to release stress and promote relaxation. The following tips and suggestions should help you get started.

Use Relaxation Exercises. The regular use of relaxation exercises can enable your body to release stored tension, and your mind to return to a natural state of balance. Many different relaxation exercises can be effective. This section presents two that many people find helpful.

To soothe muscle tension and its related stress, or to relax when you are finding it difficult to sleep, lie down in a comfortable position. Then, beginning at either your head or your toes, clench and then relax the muscles in each region of your body. For example, if you choose to start with your head, tense all of your head and facial muscles, including your jaw. Hold for a count of one or two, then let the muscles relax. Repeat the process with your neck muscles, followed in order by the muscles in your shoulders, arms, chest, abdomen, hips, thighs, calves, ankles, and feet. There is no need to strain as you perform this exercise. Simply clench and release each muscle group in turn, progressing from one end of the body to the other.

To use the second relaxation technique, sit comfortably in a quiet place with soft lightning, with your feet flat on the floor and your eyes closed. Focus your attention on your breathing, and take a few deep breaths. As you exhale, mentally tell yourself to relax. After a few minutes, become aware of the place in your body where tension might still be stored, beginning with your head, face, and jaw. Continue breathing deeply and gently, and as you exhale, visualize the tension in that area of your body passing away with your breath. As you inhale, visualize that area of the body becoming lighter and more relaxed, and feel that relaxation spreading like a wave throughout the rest of your body. Repeat this process for each part of your body in which you feel tension. When you finish, remain seated and rest quietly for a few more minutes before you open your eyes and resume your daily activities. The more you practice this exercise, the easier it will be for you to quickly trigger the "relaxation response" throughout your body.

Use Conscious Breathing. Another effective means of dispelling stress is to take deep breaths whenever you feel tension building up in your body. Typically, when you are stressed, your breathing becomes shallow, or you momentarily forget to breathe altogether. Breathing in this shallow, constricted manner only serves to exacerbate the stress you feel by limiting your intake of vital oxygen. At such times, simply taking a few minutes to breathe fully, inhaling deep inside your diaphragm, can quickly counteract stress and leave you feeling more alert and energized. The more conscious you become of your breathing patterns, the more quickly you will sense the effects of stress in your body and be able to eliminate them.

Practice Meditation. Since the 1970s, numerous studies have shown the health benefits of meditation. One of the pioneering researchers in this regard was Herbert Benson, MD, of Harvard Medical School, who coined the phrase *relaxation response*. Dr. Benson's research proved that meditation not only triggers the relaxation response, but also increases oxygen intake, increases blood flow, enhances immunity, and creates more relaxed brain-wave rhythms. In 1984, the National Institutes of Health recommended meditation over prescription drugs as a more appropriate treatment for mild hypertension.

Many schools of meditation exist, ranging from Transcendental Meditation (TM) to mindfulness meditation. While it can be very beneficial to receive meditation training from a skilled instructor, it is not necessary to do so in order to gain meditation's many health benefits. As Dr. Benson and others have shown, the same benefits can be gained simply by spending twenty to thirty minutes once or twice a day sitting comfortably, with your eyes closed, as you focus your attention on your breathing. As you do so, you may find it helpful to mentally repeat a phrase such as "peace" or "relax" each time you inhale and exhale. Don't be surprised if at first you find yourself unable to sit still for more than a few minutes. This is normal. But with commitment, you will soon find yourself able to meditate comfortably for longer periods of time. Before long, as you start to more fully experience the benefits of meditation, you will look forward to it each day.

Examine Your Beliefs and Attitudes. The way in which we cope with stressful events and stimuli is determined to a large extent by the way in which we interpret them. For example, consider two men who are cut off by another driver during morning rush hour traffic. For one man, the event might be cause for anger that he carries with him for the remainder of the day. But the other man may lightly shrug off the event as a normal part of commuting, and not give it a thought after it has passed. The men experienced similar events, but their different interpretations made a big difference in the way they felt afterwards.

Although it is certainly easier said than actually lived, we always have a choice as to how we respond to the events of the day. Therefore, in times of upset, it can be extremely helpful to remember that you are *choosing* to react in that manner. Often, simply admitting this to yourself will be all that you need to quickly let go of your feelings of distress. But in order to cultivate this habit, it is necessary to first take time to examine your habitual beliefs and attitudes, since they are usually what most influences your reaction to stressful situations.

Consider the type of person you are. Are you a person who sees the glass half full or half empty? Are you generally an optimist who believes in and expects good things in your life, or are you habitually pessimistic, believing that you have to struggle for everything you achieve in a "dog-eat-dog" world? People who are optimistic and possess positive attitudes typically do a much better job of coping with stress than people whose attitudes and beliefs are negative and pessimistic.

Fortunately, our attitudes and beliefs are not set in stone. Researchers such as Martin Seligman, PhD, author of *Learned Optimism*, have found that anyone can alter his or her beliefs and attitudes for the better, resulting in a more positive, less stressful experience of life. The first step in doing so, however, involves honest self-reflection and appraisal of what we believe, think, and feel. It has been said, "The unexamined life is not worth living." I would add that the unexamined life is often far more difficult and stressful than it needs to be.

Take the time to examine your core attitudes and beliefs. You can easily do this by keeping a journal or by simply listing your responses to important life issues. You may be surprised to discover how little evidence actually exists to support those beliefs and attitudes that do not serve you. After making such discoveries, you can then do something about them. You can substitute more positive attitudes and beliefs for those you wish to discard, and you can dramatically change your life for the better.

Cultivate a Sense of Humor. The ability to perceive humor in the situations in which you find yourself, and the ability to laugh, can be a powerful antidote to stress. The Bible says, "A cheerful heart is good medicine." Two researchers who have explored the health benefits of humor are Robert Ornstein, PhD, and David Sobel, MD, authors of *Healthy Pleasures*. They write, "A robust laugh gives the muscles of your face, shoulders, diaphragm, and abdomen a good workout. With convulsive or side-splitting laughter, even your arm and leg muscles come into play. Your heart rate and blood pressure temporarily rise, breathing becomes faster and deeper, and oxygen surges through your bloodstream. . . . The afterglow of a hearty laugh is positively relaxing. Blood pressure may temporarily fall, your muscles go limp, and you bask in a mild euphoria."

Studies have also shown that laughter can boost immunity, as well as dissipate the effects of stress. Moreover, laughter and a positive sense of humor foster other positive attitudes and beliefs. If you want to incorporate more humor and laughter in your life, consider the following suggestions:

❑ Make it a habit to rent a comic movie or a taped comedy routine at least once a week. There are dozens and dozens of classic old movies that are guaranteed to do the job.

❑ Read humorous books that show the funny side of life.

❑ Spend less time with people who are depressing and pessimistic, and more time with people with whom you can share laughter. As obvious as this seems, you would be surprised by how few of us consider this option. Once you connect with people who are happy, you'll quickly see that laughter is infectious.

❑ Get yourself on a few funny e-mail lists. One word of caution here: Make sure you have an up-to-date anti-virus software program loaded in your computer.

By making a conscious effort to add humor to your life, you will find yourself enjoying your life more fully. You will also minimize stress and improve your overall health.

CONCLUSION

As this chapter makes clear, there are specific key factors that you must control if you are to make a successful journey to optimal health. By incorporating the recommendations made in this chapter into your daily life, you will soon notice significant improvements in your health. But there is another element of optimal health—the pH Factor. By understanding and taking control of this factor, you will truly gain control of your life and your well-being. Chapter 3 will fill you in on the details.

3

The pH Factor

balanced pH is one of the most vital components of good health. Too often, however, doctors ignore acid-alkaline balance—a mistake that can potentially lead to serious health problems. In this chapter, you will learn why the pH Factor is so important to your health, and you will discover how an unbalanced pH can lead to disease. You will also learn how to determine the state of your own pH Factor. Is your body in balance? Are you too acidic? Are you too alkaline? Let's begin by learning more about what pH and acid-alkaline balance really are.

WHAT IS THE pH FACTOR?

As you learned in Chapter 1, pH refers to the relative concentration of hydrogen ions in a solution such as blood, urine, or saliva. The term itself was first defined in 1909 by a Danish biochemist named Soren Peter Lauritz Sorensen. Since that time, it has been used to measure the acidic, alkaline, or neutral properties of various solutions and compounds. In terms of health, pH is a measurement of the acid-alkaline ratio of the body's fluids and tissues. When this ratio is in balance, good health results. When it is out of balance—either too acidic or too alkaline—the body's internal environment is negatively affected, setting the stage for disease.

pH is measured on a scale of 0 to 14. A pH of 7 is considered neutral, while values below 7 show a greater concentration of positively charged hydrogen ions compared to negatively charged ions. Conversely, a pH value greater than 7 indicates a higher concentration of negatively charged ions. A pH reading below 7 is an indication of acidity, and a reading above 7 indicates an alkaline condition.

pH, Acids, and Hydrogen Ions in the Body

All acids in the body contain hydrogen molecules. *Molecule* is the term we use to denote the smallest particle into which an element or compound can be divided without losing any of its characteristics. The smallest molecular structures consist of a single atom, while a combination of two or more atoms creates molecular chemical compounds, including hydrogen. When hydrogen molecules are dissolved in water—a process known as *dissociation*—they create hydrogen ions. Hydrogen ions are single, unstable protons that literally "hide" in the body's water molecules.

All acids in the body give off hydrogen ions when they are dissolved in water. In fact, this very property is what makes these substances acids. Any substance that reacts with acids is known as a *base,* and any base that dissolves in water is known as an *alkali.* Whether a substance is acidic or alkaline depends on the concentration of ions within it. The measurement of this concentration is called "potential for hydrogen," or pH for short. The pH scale of measurement ranges from 0 to 14, with 7 being neutral—neither acidic or alkaline. Any measurement below 7 is considered acidic, while any measurement above 7 is considered alkaline. The greater the concentration of hydrogen ions in a substance, the more acidic it is.

pH values are determined according to the concentration of hydrogen ions represented as moles per liter. (The term *mole* is short for *molecular weight.*) Pure water, which is considered neutral, has a concentration of hydrogen ions that equals 0.0000001 moles per liter, or 10^{-7} moles per liter. By contrast, an extremely acidic substance might have a concentration of hydrogen ions as high as 0.01, or 10^{-2} moles per liter.

As you can see from these examples, concentrations of hydrogen ions are written as a power of 10. To indicate their pH values, we simply remove the base number 10 and the minus sign. Thus, a pH of 7 would be the value of pure (neutral) water, while a pH of 2 would indicate very high acidity. An increase of one point of pH is equal to a tenfold *decrease* in hydrogen ion concentration, while a decrease of one point of pH equals a ten-fold *increase* in hydrogen ion concentration.

Your body can thrive only when your blood chemistry is slightly alkaline. As you saw in Chapter 1, for a state of optimal health to exist, the pH of your blood should be 7.365. When your pH blood reading moves too far below or above this number and remains that way, the inevitable result is illness. Some people who are chronically ill have a blood pH that is overly alkaline. However, in my clinical experience, I have found that the majority of people suffering from chronic illness have a blood pH that is far too acidic.

When this state of over-acidity becomes chronic, a number of serious health threats can arise. This occurs because the bloodstream environment diminishes the body's internal oxygen supply and supports disease-producing microorganisms. We will discuss these factors in more detail later in this chapter. First, though, I want to point out that not all parts of the body operate within the same pH range. This is because, as Dr. Arthur Guyton explains in his *Textbook of Medical Physiology,* there are different levels of acidity and alkalinity in which your body's various organs, tissues, and fluids can function optimally. Examples of Dr. Guyton's findings are shown in Table 3.1, which lists various body organs, tissues, and fluids and their respective pH range. In each of these areas, a particular pH range is necessary for the numerous chemical and enzyme reactions to occur. Small changes in pH levels can profoundly affect the body's overall function and energy levels.

TABLE 3.1. HEALTHY pH VALUES OF THE HUMAN BODY			
BODY FLUIDS, TISSUES, AND ORGANS	HEALTHY pH VALUE	BODY FLUIDS, TISSUES, AND ORGANS	HEALTHY pH VALUE
Blood	7.35–7.45	Saliva	6.0–7.4
Brain	7.1	Skeletal Muscle	6.9–7.2
Heart	7.0–7.4	Skin	5.4–5.9
Liver	7.2	Urine	4.5–8.0

As you can see from this table, the pH of both saliva and urine can vary fairly widely without compromising the overall health of the body. Blood pH, on the other hand, must remain within a much narrower range. This is why I believe that the blood pH reading is the most important determinant of your body's acid-alkaline balance.

HOW THE BODY REGULATES PH

Because appropriate pH levels are so vital to maintaining proper
body function, nature has designed a number of interrelated mechanisms that help regulate the acid-alkaline balance of the body's fluids, organs, and tissues. These mechanisms work in two ways. They
either eliminate excess acid, or they neutralize acid by drawing upon
the body's mineral stores. Let's examine how each of these self-regulating processes work.

Eliminating Acids

The elimination of acids is chiefly accomplished by the kidneys and
lungs, and to a lesser extent, by the skin. Your kidneys play a vital

Sodium's Influence on Health and Illness

In proper concentrations, the mineral sodium plays an essential role in
the maintenance of good health. Found primarily in the blood and in the
fluids inside and around the cells, sodium is vital for normal nerve and
muscle function, and is required to maintain normal fluid balance within the body. When sodium levels become too high or too low, however,
imbalances can result, setting the stage for disease.

Your body's supply of sodium is derived from the foods and drinks
you consume, while sodium is excreted primarily through perspiration
and urination. Your kidneys seek to maintain a consistent level of sodium
in the body by regulating the amount of sodium that is eliminated. But
when sodium intake and excretion are not in balance, the total amount of
sodium in the body is affected. Changes in your body's sodium levels
directly affect your body's blood volume—that is, the amount of water
found in your bloodstream. Too little sodium causes blood volume to
decrease, while too much sodium causes blood volume to increase.

Your body continually monitors blood volume via sensors in the
heart, blood vessels, and kidneys. When blood volume becomes too high,
your kidneys attempt to increase sodium excretion in order to return blood
volume levels to normal. When blood volume starts to become low, your
body's adrenal and pituitary glands secrete hormones that cause your kidneys to retain both sodium and water in order to increase blood volume.

Low blood sodium levels occur when your body's sodium supply becomes over-diluted. This can be caused by drinking excessive amounts of water or by receiving water intravenously in above-normal amounts during hospitalization. Heart failure, cirrhosis of the liver, kidney problems, chronic diarrhea, and improper secretion of hormones by the pituitary or adrenal glands can also deplete blood sodium levels. Other causes include excessive exercise and/or perspiration, infection, and the use of diuretic medications.

Low blood sodium levels particularly affect the brain, which is highly sensitive to changes in sodium levels. As the brain becomes affected, you may feel yourself becoming lethargic, confused, or lightheaded. If the condition worsens, additional symptoms, including muscle twitching and seizures, can also occur. In severe cases of low blood sodium levels, the result can be stupor, coma, and even death. Determining the cause of low blood sodium levels is difficult and requires a complete diagnostic checkup by a physician. If the condition is found to exist, you will be advised to restrict your fluid intake to no more than one quart per day. In severe cases, additional medical intervention may be required.

The more common form of sodium imbalance is high blood sodium levels. When this occurs, your body lacks enough water to cope with the amount of sodium it contains. The primary cause of high blood sodium levels is dehydration, a common condition in the United States due to the fact that most people fail to drink enough water each day, and also eat foods that are high in sodium. Other possible causes include diarrhea, vomiting, fever, excessive sweating (particularly during hot weather), abnormal kidney function, diabetes, head trauma or surgery involving the pituitary gland, imbalanced calcium and/or potassium levels, sickle cell anemia, and use of drugs such as corticosteroids or diuretics.

The most common symptoms of high blood sodium levels are confusion, depression, fatigue, fluid retention, irritability, lack of coordination, muscle cramps or twitching, nausea, restlessness, and general weakness. More serious symptoms can include changes in blood pressure and heart rate, coma, seizure, and death. A checkup by your physician is necessary to determine if you suffer from high blood sodium levels. To treat the condition, you will be advised to avoid salty foods and salty liquids, such as sports drinks, and to increase your intake of water.

role in the regulation of blood pH by helping to eliminate what are known as fixed or solid acids, such as uric and sulfuric acids. When pH levels become too acidic, the kidneys excrete additional hydrogen ions into the urine, while retaining extra sodium. This process filters fixed acids out of the bloodstream, diluting them so that they can be eliminated in the urine. Phosphate—a form of the mineral phosphorus—is required for this to occur, and if enough reserves are not available, the body draws phosphorus directly from its bones.

In cases of extreme acidity, the kidneys excrete aluminum ions, which contain four types of hydrogen, into the urine. But the kidneys are able to eliminate only a set amount of acids each day, no matter how hard they work. When the buildup of fixed acids exceeds the kidneys' maximum daily capacity for elimination, problems can occur. Signs that your body is too acidic include cloudy and/or rust-colored urine, and a noticeable urine odor. When acidic buildup is particularly high, a burning sensation can also accompany urination. It's important to note, however, that changes in urine color and odor can also be due to other factors, including various disease conditions. (See the inset on page 45 to learn more about the meaning of urine color and odor.)

As you breathe, your lungs also help regulate acid-alkaline balance. During respiration, carbon dioxide combines with water in the blood to form a type of acid called carbonic acid. Respiration helps remove carbonic acid from the bloodstream, thus decreasing acidity. Your rate of respiration varies, depending on how acidic or alkaline your body is. In conditions of over-acidity, your respiratory rate will tend to become faster as your body attempts to remove higher levels of carbonic acid and help bring acid-alkaline levels back into balance. In conditions of excess alkalinity, respiration rates tend to slow down as the body seeks to retain the acids needed to reduce alkaline levels.

The sweat glands in your skin also help eliminate acids. As you perspire, acids are flushed out of your body. However, less acids are eliminated in this process than in urination. On average, you eliminate nearly one quart of sweat every twenty-four hours, compared with the one and a half quarts of urine eliminated during the same period. In addition, smaller concentrations of acids are carried away by sweat than by urine. Strong-smelling perspiration is usually an indication that your body is too acidic.

Possible Indications of Changes in Urine Color and Odor

While changes in urine color and odor can often accompany excessive acid buildup in the body, such changes can also be due to other conditions. Some of these conditions are relatively benign. For instance, an unusual odor can be caused by dehydration, infection, or the overconsumption of nutritional supplements, especially the B vitamins. Even certain foods can create this condition. Asparagus, for instance, are notorious for producing urine odor, especially among people who don't usually eat them. But strong urine odor can also be caused by underlying illnesses, including diabetes, kidney stones, and urinary tract infections.

Changes in urine color can also be due to dehydration, particularly if the urine is cloudy or rust-colored. Urine color change can also result from overexercise or exertion; eating certain foods, such as asparagus, beets, blackberries, borscht, or rhubarb; taking nutritional supplements, which can cause urine to become bright yellow or orange; or using medications, including laxatives. A change can also be caused by blood in the urine or by various disease conditions, including bladder cancer, cervical cancer, cirrhosis of the liver, diabetes, diarrhea, enlarged prostate (BPH), gonorrhea, hepatitis (A, B, or C), jaundice, kidney cancer, kidney disease, kidney stones, pancreatic cancer, prostate cancer, prostatitis (prostate infection), tuberculosis, urinary stones, or urinary tract infections. If changes in urine odor or color persist or are accompanied by other symptoms, the best course of action is to seek prompt medical attention.

Neutralizing Acid Buildup

Neutralization of acids occurs both during the digestive process and through cellular metabolism. When you eat a meal, as the foods you consume are digested, both the stomach and pancreas secrete substances that can affect acid-alkaline balance. As these secretions are absorbed into the bloodstream during digestion, they are then circulated throughout the rest of the body. The stomach secretes hydrochloric acid (HCl) to help the body break down food. This, in turn, causes the pancreas to secrete bicarbonate, a form of acid salt that neutralizes, or buffers, HCl after it has performed its function. If HCl is not neutralized, it can interfere with the pancreatic enzymes that are also necessary for proper digestion.

Usually, these secretions create temporary changes in blood pH called acid and alkaline tides. But once the digestive process is complete, blood pH returns to normal. However, poor diet as well as the other factors discussed in Chapter 2 can interfere with this process, causing these secretions to become unbalanced. This can create havoc in the body. (See the inset below to learn about one of the most common results of acid-alkaline imbalance.)

Heartburn

On the text presented above, you learned that poor diet and other factors can cause an acid-alkaline imbalance. One of the most common symptoms of this imbalance is heartburn, which occurs when small amounts of acid rise into the esophagus. Many people take heartburn medications—Tums, Rolaids, and the like—to deal with the discomfort caused by this condition. But although these medications offer temporary relief, they do not address the underlying cause of heartburn. In fact, studies indicate that when these antacids are used on a regular basis, they can actually make the problem worse by disrupting the body's acid-alkaline balance. Ultimately, these drugs can interfere with your body's ability to properly absorb folic acid, vitamin B^{12}, and many of the minerals essential for good health.

Ironically, the many television ads you see for heartburn medications imply that heartburn is due to excess production of stomach acid (HCl). In actuality, this isn't true. Research published as early as the 1960s, in peer-reviewed medical journals such as *Lancet,* indicated that in most cases of abnormal HCl production, *too little* HCl is being produced, not *too much.* This is especially true as we get older. When HCl is lacking, certain foods, especially proteins, are only partially digested, which can lead to the fermentation of undigested food particles in the stomach, resulting in mucus buildup along the intestinal tract—and a host of problems. Fortunately, in the vast majority of cases, when dietary habits improve, heartburn and other digestion-related issues are automatically resolved.

Mechanisms designed to regulate the acid-alkaline balance are also present within each individual cell, where balance is primarily maintained in two ways. In the first method, regulation is achieved by pumps within the cell membrane. It is through these pumps that hydrogen molecules enter and exit the cells. In the second method, internal cellular pH levels are maintained by the cells themselves, which alter chemical reactions depending on how much or how little hydrogen needs to be produced.

When pH imbalances are prolonged, the body will seek to compensate for them by drawing out various minerals—including calcium, magnesium, potassium, and sodium—from bones and organs. It does so in order to neutralize the buildup of acids and then safely eliminate them. But when the body has to resort to such methods for long periods, it places itself under internal strain. Such stress can eventually create great damage to the body, causing premature aging, excessive weight gain, lack of energy, and impaired digestion and elimination, among a host of other conditions. The most common conditions and side effects caused by lengthy imbalances are discussed below, as well as in Chapter 4.

THE HARMFUL EFFECTS OF pH IMBALANCES

As you have seen, when pH levels become imbalanced for prolonged periods of time, your body's internal environment becomes either too acidic or too alkaline. In the vast majority of cases, over-acidity, or *acidosis*, is the problem. Many health practitioners who address pH imbalance focus only on acidosis because of the high incidence with which this condition occurs. But for some people, over-alkalinity, also known as *alkalosis*, is at the heart of their health problems.

Alkalosis

Although conditions of alkalosis are far rarer than acidosis, they too can cause various health problems. According to Dr. Arthur Guyton, alkalosis is primarily caused by the overconsumption of drugs that produce an alkalizing effect in the body, especially the antiheartburn preparations discussed previously, as well as prescribed ulcer medications. Alkalosis can also occur as a result of chronic diarrhea or vomiting, both of which can cause the loss of HCl and other acids. When alkalosis sets in, your body is deprived of the acids that are necessary to maintain proper balance.

The major side effect of alkalosis is overexcitability of the nervous system. According to Dr. Guyton, "This effect occurs both in the central nervous system and in the peripheral nerves [all nerves located outside of the central nervous system], but usually the peripheral nerves are affected before the central nervous system. The nerves become so excitable that they automatically and repetitively fire even when they are not stimulated by normal stimuli." This, in turn, can lead to a condition known as *tetany*, a painful disorder characterized by muscle spasm and/or muscle cramps. Interestingly, tetany can also be caused by hyperventilation, or "overbreathing." As you learned earlier in this chapter, breathing is one of the ways that your body rids itself of excess acids. When we hyperventilate, too many acids can be eliminated, leading both to tetany and to a temporary state of alkalosis.

If the peripheral nerves continue to be affected by alkalosis, eventually the central nervous system can become affected as well. Although the likelihood of this happening is not great, when it does occur, the consequences can be serious. The most common symptom is extreme nervousness due to the overstimulation of the central nervous system itself. In acute cases, convulsions can also occur. People who suffer from epilepsy can experience seizures if their bodies become too alkaline. Such people would do well to avoid alkaline drugs, or to use them only under the strict supervision of their physician. The dietary suggestions in Chapter 5 can also be beneficial.

Acidosis—The Primary Culprit

As I've stated, the majority of pH imbalances are related to acidosis, caused by an excess of acids in the body's internal environment. When acid buildup occurs to the point where the body is no longer able to successfully eliminate or neutralize these acids, a host of problems can occur, including accelerated aging, demineralization, fatigue, impaired enzyme activity, inflammation and organ damage, and the proliferation of harmful microorganisms such as bacteria, fungi, molds, yeasts, and viruses. Let's examine each of these problems in turn.

Accelerated Aging

Accelerated or premature aging is all too common in our society. This condition can be caused by a variety of factors, such as the accumulation of environmental toxins in the body, stress, and nutritional deficiencies. As we saw in Chapter 2, these factors can also affect pH levels, making your body more susceptible to disease. When your body's cells are continually exposed to an overly acidic environment, their cell structure can become altered, meaning that the cells walls lose their integrity. When viewed under a microscope, such cells, instead of being round and having noticeably strong walls, look bent and misshapen, with cell walls that are thin and weak. In addition, their ability to function properly can be diminished, as can their ability to effectively communicate with other cells. Over time, this state of deterioration causes the cells to make "mistakes" as they seek to repair and regenerate themselves by manufacturing essential proteins.

Heat shock protein, a substance required by your body to facilitate cellular repair, is one of the many proteins that can be affected by acidosis. This protein is important as it aids in the disposal of old or damaged proteins while helping to build and transport new proteins. Acidosis impairs your body's ability to produce this substance, thereby hampering the process of cellular repair. This, in turn, can trigger premature cell death as a result of the wrong proteins being manufactured, or of the right proteins being manufactured in inadequate amounts. When this happens, shortages of substances such as collagen and elastin—both of which are essential for healthy, wrinkle-free, young-looking skin—can arise, as well as impairment of your body's internal organ systems.

Acidosis can also impair proper brain function, which is associated with aging. An overly acidic internal environment inhibits function of the *neurons*—the specialized nerve cells that conduct impulses, allowing the brain to learn, reason, and remember. When neurons are unable to function properly, symptoms such as "brain fog," forgetfulness, and impaired mental acuity are more apt to occur.

Demineralization

As already discussed, your body draws upon its alkaline mineral stores in order to buffer or neutralize excess acids. While occasional withdrawal of these minerals is not likely to pose a problem, during chronic acidosis, the loss of such minerals—which include calcium, potassium, magnesium, and sodium—can pose serious health risks. Since these minerals are stored in all body tissues, their loss can potentially affect any of your body's organs. But it is your bones and teeth that are most affected by demineralization.

Dr. Susan E. Brown is a world-renowned expert in *osteoporosis*—a disease in which the bones become extremely porous. Dr. Brown points out that this condition is virtually nonexistent in cultures around the world that traditionally eat whole foods, which help foster a balanced pH. In her book *Better Bones, Better Body*, she states, "In our society, we consume a very imbalanced diet high in acid-forming foods. This imbalanced diet pushes us towards an acid state. . . . [E]xcessive and prolonged acidity can drain bone of calcium reserves and lead to bone thinning." As this thinning process occurs, your bones lose their flexibility, increasing the risk of osteoporosis. You become far more susceptible to age-related fractures, such as hip, wrist, and forearm fractures; to rheumatism; and to degeneration of the spinal disks, potentially leading to conditions such as chronic back pain and sciatica.

Demineralization can also lead to tooth problems, since loss of calcium makes teeth more brittle and more susceptible to chipping. Your teeth may also start to experience sensitivity to hot and cold foods, and be more prone to develop cavities. Tooth decay and cavities, so prevalent in children today, are almost always caused by a steady diet of acid-forming foods, such as sugared cereals, sodas, and fast-food meals. Other common results of demineralization include dry and cracking skin, brittle and thinning hair, fingernails that crack or split easily, and gums that are oversensitive and bleed easily.

Fatigue

In my practice, I've found that fatigue is one of the most common symptoms among people whose bodies have become overly acidic. As over-acidity grows worse, so, too, does fatigue. The reason for this is fairly simple and straightforward. Acidosis creates an internal environment that is not conducive to optimal energy production.

In an overly acidic environment, your body's blood supply of oxygen diminishes, making oxygen less available to the cells, tissues, and organs, and thereby interfering with cell repair. Lack of oxygen also impairs the ability of the mitochondria—your cell's internal "energy factories"—to function. When the mitochondria are not well protected and properly fed—both consequences of acidosis and diminished oxygen supply—their ability to communicate with one another breaks down. This, in turns, compromises the mitochondria's energy production, leading to fatigue.

In an *anaerobic* (low oxygen) environment, toxins and harmful microorganisms are also better able to flourish and proliferate. As they do so, they interfere with the body's ability to absorb and utilize nutrients. This malabsorption of nutrients makes it much more difficult for your body to manufacture the enzymes, hormones, and numerous other biochemical substances required for energy production, proper organ activity, and cellular repair. Blood sugar levels can also be affected, further impairing physical endurance.

The growth of microorganisms such as yeasts and fungus can also disturb the balance of *electrolytes*—minerals that act as conductors of electricity throughout the body and play a vital role in cellular activity. When electrolytes become imbalanced, the normal flow of energy in the body is reduced. If all of these factors are left unchecked, the result is chronic fatigue. This explains why people who suffer from chronic fatigue syndrome (CFS) invariably also suffer from acidosis. In my experience, acidosis comes first, and leads to CFS. By understanding acidosis, treating it, and resolving it, you can also free yourself from fatigue.

Impaired Enzyme Activity

According to Edward Howell, MD, author of *Enzyme Nutrition,* "Enzymes are substances that make life possible. No mineral, vitamin, or hormone can do any work without enzymes. They are the manual workers that build the body from proteins, carbohydrates, and fats. The body may have the raw building materials, but without the workers it cannot begin."

Thousands of different types of enzymes are manufactured by the body. Each one of them acts as a specific biological catalyst, stimulating a particular biochemical reaction. Enzymes are necessary for every single process that the body performs, including breathing, digestion, immune function, reproduction, and proper organ function, as well as speech, thought, and movement. But enzymes can perform their multitude of tasks only within specific pH levels.

When pH levels become imbalanced, as they do in the case of acidosis, enzyme function becomes disrupted. In some instances, enzyme activity can cease altogether as a result of unhealthy pH levels. When this happens, illness occurs. Initially, the illness will usually be mild in nature, but it can quickly become more severe if the body's proper acid-alkaline balance is not restored. If enzyme function is completely shut down due to unhealthy pH levels, death will eventually ensue.

Many of my holistic colleagues recommend supplementing the diet with digestive and metabolic enzymes in order to guard against such health-sapping effects. For some people, this is absolutely vital. Overall, however, enzyme supplementation will not achieve lasting results as long as the body remains in a state of chronic acidosis. Since over-acidity is the underlying cause of enzyme malfunction, it makes far better sense to restore the internal environment to its proper acid-alkaline balance.

Inflammation and Organ Damage

When the body has an overly acidic pH, the excess acids—which are highly corrosive—can be damaging to the tissues and organs with which they come in contact. If not neutralized or eliminated, they can cause lesions and hardening of organ tissues, as well as inflammation. The kidneys and skin—both organs through which acids are eliminated—can be particularly affected when the amount of acid is too great for these organs to handle. When the skin is affected, conditions such as hives, eczema, blotching, and itching can occur as a direct result of acidic sweat passing through the sweat glands. When excess acid buildup occurs in the kidneys, the urinary tract can become inflamed, causing a painful, burning sensation during urination. Infection can also occur, leading to conditions such as cystitis, a type of bladder inflammation that is often accompanied by urinary tract infection.

Inflammation caused by acid buildup can occur anywhere in the body, leading to illnesses ending with "-itis"—a suffix used to indicate an inflammatory condition. Inflammation of the joints can cause arthritis, for example, while inflammation of the nerves can lead to neuritis, and inflammation in the lungs can cause bronchitis. Inflammation of the gastrointestinal tract can result in colitis or enteritis.

Compounding this problem is the fact that acid buildup also impairs immune function. In a state of acidosis, production of white blood cells is diminished, and the white blood cells that are manufactured are of reduced strength. Since white blood cells play a vital role in the body's ability to target and destroy invading microbes, their diminished numbers and capacity resulting from excess acids in the body makes it easier for disease to take hold.

Proliferation of Harmful Microorganisms

When the pH of the blood remains consistently below 7.365, the bloodstream becomes a breeding ground for harmful microorganisms, much like a stagnant swamp. This happens because acidosis reduces the available oxygen supply in the bloodstream, and microorganisms thrive in the absence of optimum oxygen levels.

Bacteria, fungi, molds, yeasts, and viruses subsist by fermenting glucose, which under healthy conditions is used by your body to supply energy. In addition, they take the fats and proteins normally used by your body for regeneration and other functions, and use them instead for their own reproduction. In this way, the microorganisms are able to spread throughout the body, targeting weak areas, breaking down tissue, and interfering with bodily processes that are essential for good health.

The most serious health problem posed by microorganisms is not the microorganisms themselves, but the waste products they produce during their life cycle. These excretions are also acidic. As they are dumped into your bloodstream, they further pollute your internal environment and invade your cells, to directly or indirectly produce a wide range of disease symptoms, all of which worsen as the microorganisms continue to proliferate. Among the more common of these symptoms are:

❑ Allergies, including chemical sensitivities, food allergies, food craving, and hay fever.

❑ Bladder and urinary tract infections.

❑ Bleeding and/or receding gums.

❑ Candidiasis.

❑ Colds and flu.

❑ Cysts.

❑ Dizziness.

❑ Dry mouth.

❑ Endometriosis.

❑ Finger and/or toenail fungus.

❑ Gastrointestinal disorders, including acid reflux, bloating, colitis, constipation, diarrhea, enteritis, flatulence, halitosis, heartburn, hemorrhoids, indigestion, intestinal pains, and ulcers.

❑ Headache.

❑ Hormonal imbalances, including adrenal and thyroid dysfunction.

❑ Hypoglycemia (low blood sugar).

❑ Hyperactivity.

❑ Impaired immunity and greater susceptibility to infectious disease.

❑ Joint pain and/or muscle ache.

❑ Low libido, including lessened sex drive, ambition, and joy.

❑ Mental and emotional disorders, including antisocial behavior, anxiety, depression, irritability, mood swings, poor memory, and suicidal tendencies.

❑ PMS and menstrual problems.

❑ Skin problems, including dry skin, hives, itching, and skin rash.

❑ Sleep disorders.

❑ Weight problems, including excessive weight gain or unhealthy weight loss.

DETERMINING YOUR PH

Now that you understand the importance of pH to your health, you might wish to know your own pH levels. While there are a number of tests available for measuring pH levels in the body, let's focus on two testing procedures. The first is the venous plasma pH test, which can provide you with an accurate reading of your blood's pH level. The second is a self-test that can be easily performed at home. Although the self-test does not provide specific pH measurements, through the use of pH strips, it does offer a strong indication of your acidic-alkaline balance.

The Venous Plasma pH Test

The venous plasma pH test accurately measures the pH of your blood. The test must be administered by a physician, who will withdraw a vial of bottle from the vein in your arm, and then send the blood to a licensed laboratory for testing. Should you decide to have this test performed, be sure to request that the measurement be made to the nearest one-hundredth of a percentage point—for example, 7.36 or 7.25, not 7.3 or 7.2. This will provide a more precise reading of your blood pH.

Because blood pH levels are so important to your overall health, I recommend that you make the venous plasma pH test part of your annual physical checkup. Since it is not commonly administered as part of such checkups, be sure to ask your physician for it when you schedule your appointment. The additional cost is nominal—usually less than $100—and the information the test provides can literally save your life.

The pH Strip

Although I have emphasized the importance of blood pH—a factor that can be measured only by laboratory testing—you can also perform a simple home pH test using pH strips, which are usually available in drugstores as well as some health food stores. pH strips are made of litmus paper, which changes color when it comes in contact with alkaline and acidic substances. Included with your purchase will be a color chart that will help you to gauge your pH.

When you perform the test, the strip will turn one of three colors: yellow, which indicates over-acidity; blue or red (depending on the manufacturer of the strips), which indicates over-alkalinity; or green, which indicates a neutral or balanced pH reading. The intensity of the color is important. The deeper or more intense the shade, the more extreme the pH reading. For example, a light yellow shade is an indication of less serious over-acidity, while a deep shade of yellow indicates a more serious problem. In actuality, both shadings indicate that the pH is out of balance and overly acidic, but the deeper shade of yellow is a sign of a more serious imbalance.

You can use pH strips to test the pH levels of both your urine and your saliva. However, I recommend testing your urine instead. As mentioned earlier, your kidneys are one of the organs used by the body to eliminate acids. When your body is in or near a state of acid-alkaline balance, urine pH will normally be 7.0 to 7.5. (pH strips do not measure pH values as closely as a blood pH test does.) This indicates that your kidneys are excreting normal levels of acids. But when higher-than-normal amounts of acids are being eliminated, it means that your body is overly acidic. Similarly, if lower-than-normal levels of acids are being excreted, it means that your body is overly alkaline.

Since urine pH values can change during the day in reaction to the foods you eat, the best time to measure urine pH is in the morning soon after you've awakened, before you've had your morning meal. It is easy to perform the test. Simply take a pH strip and quickly dip it into your urine stream as you urinate. As the acid content of your urine reacts with the pH strip, it will change color.

Remember that a urine pH test does not provide a truly accurate indication of your body's internal acid-alkaline balance, but it can help you get a sense of your body's internal environment. I recommend that you perform this test for five mornings in a row. If your reading is consistently within the range of 7.0 to 7.5, you can feel confident that your body is in a fairly healthy state of acid-alkaline balance. Consistent readings below 7.0 indicate over-acidity.

Interestingly, consistent readings above 7.5 do not necessarily mean that your body is overly alkaline. Several pH readings above 7.5 can mean one of three things. The first possibility is that your body's internal environment is in a healthy state of acid-alkaline balance or is only slightly alkaline. This is likely to be the case if you regularly consume foods that have an alkalizing effect on the body, and if you limit your consumption of acid-producing foods, such as meats and dairy products. (More information about both classes of foods is provided in Chapter 5.) Or the reading could be due to the ingestion of alkaline mineral supplements that your body has little use for. In this first case, a urine pH reading above 7.5 does not indicate imbalance or disease. Nonetheless, some precautions are advisable. For example, if you are following a vegetarian diet, you should be careful to avoid dietary deficiencies that can be caused by lack of protein from animal products. If you are supplementing with alkalizing supplements, it might be advisable to reduce your intake or to stop taking the supplements altogether.

The second possibility for urine pH readings consistently above 7.5 is far more serious. If you are not following an alkalizing diet or taking alkalizing supplements, such high readings could indicate an imbalance in your endocrine system, which governs the manufacture and regulation of hormones. In particular, a higher pH reading might indicate adrenal or parathyroid gland problems. Or it could be an indication that another form of illness is present. Although such occurrences are rare, it would be wise to consult with your physician to determine if you are at risk for such problems.

In what might seem to be a paradox, the third possibility for consistently high pH readings is that your body is, in fact, acidic. How is this possible? You will recall that your kidneys can eliminate only a certain amount of acids each day. Once this capacity is met, excess acid stores start to accumulate in your body, forcing it to draw upon its alkaline reserves. Residues of these alkaline minerals get deposited in the urine, causing high pH readings. If this is the case, it is vital that you do all you can to restore your body's internal acid-alkaline balance, because you are most likely on the road to disease.

This third scenario is actually fairly common in our society. To help you better determine if you fall into this category, you'll want to consider if you are also suffering from one of the symptoms of chronic acidosis. If you are experiencing only one or two such symptoms, your body is not necessarily too acidic, but if more than a few symptoms are present, most likely you fall into this third category. The most common symptoms of acidosis are the following:

❑ Bladder and urinary tract problems, including a burning sensation during urination, excessive urination, and kidney stones.

❑ Circulatory problems, including poor circulation, hypotension (low blood pressure), feelings of coldness in the extremities, and rapid heartbeat.

❑ Energy level problems, including chronic fatigue, lack of energy, long recovery time after physical or mental exertion, loss of endurance, fatigue after eating meals, chills and/or low body temperature, and increased tendency to catch infections.

❑ Eye and facial problems, including conjunctivitis, eyes that tear easily, headache, and pale complexion caused by contracting blood vessels.

❑ Gastrointestinal problems, including abdominal pains or cramping, acid reflux, burning sensation in the anus or rectum, diarrhea, flatulence, stomach pains or spasms, and ulcers.

❑ Mental and emotional problems, including feelings of agitation or nervousness, anxiety, depression, feelings of being overwhelmed, frequent feelings of stress, irritability, lack of ambition, and lack of joy.

❏ Mouth and dental problems, including bleeding or inflamed gums, cavities, cracked lips, cracked or chipped teeth, loose teeth, mouth ulcers, tooth pain, and tooth sensitivity to hot or cold foods.

❏ Musculoskeletal problems, including "cracking" joints, muscle cramps or spasms, joint pain, muscle ache, stiff neck, and tension in the neck and shoulders.

❏ Nail and hair problems, including brittle or dull hair, hair loss, thin or splitting nails, and white spots or streaks on nails.

❏ Respiratory problems, including allergies, chronic bronchitis, frequent colds, frequent coughs or sore throat, laryngitis, runny nose, and sensitivity to cold air.

❏ Skin problems, including acne, dry skin, eczema, hives, itching, and skin blotching or red spots.

❏ Sleep problems, including insomnia or restless sleep patterns.

❏ Vaginal discharge.

If you suffer from two or more of these symptoms, there is a high probability that you are overly acidic, even if your urine pH shows a reading above 7.5. More than likely, you are also eating a diet that is too high in acid-producing foods. As you will learn in Chapter 5, by simply changing your diet so that the majority of the foods you eat are alkalizing, you can help restore your acid-alkaline balance.

CONCLUSION

By now you understand why the proper acid-alkaline balance is so important to your overall health. You have also become aware of the many symptoms that can occur when this balance is disrupted. In addition, you have learned how prolonged pH imbalances can lead to serious health problems, and even prove fatal if they are not addressed in time. Fortunately, as you will see in the following chapters, there is much that you can do to bring your body's pH levels back into balance and, in the process, regain your health.

4

Many Diseases— One Primary Cause

cientists estimate that our bodies are composed of approximately 75 trillion cells, which are divided into 150 different types. These include nerve cells, blood cells, bone cells, muscle cells, and so forth—each of which performs specialized tasks. These cell groups work with one another to govern, orchestrate, and carry out all of the body's life-sustaining functions, including self-regulation, self-repair, and self-renewal. The different groups of cells work well so long as they receive an adequate supply of oxygen, water, vitamins, minerals, enzymes, and essential fatty acids, as well as the other materials that serve as their building blocks. When this supply of nutrients is diminished or cut off, however, it sets the stage for disease and premature aging.

Once disease takes hold in the cells, it begins to attack various organs and body systems, such as the immune and endocrine systems. It is clear, then, that the health of the body depends on the health of its cells. In this chapter, you will discover the important role that proper pH balance plays in ensuring that disease does not take root. You will also take a look at our most common diseases from the unique perspective of acid-alkaline imbalance.

THE RELATIONSHIP BETWEEN PH AND CELL HEALTH

Your body's cells communicate with one another through a complex interaction of electrical, chemical, and hormonal processes. For proper communication between cells to take place, a slightly alkaline blood pH (7.365) is absolutely essential. When pH levels remain

above or below this level, cellular communication can become interrupted, and health problems can occur.

As you learned in the previous chapter, the most common type
of pH imbalance is over-acidity, or acidosis. The acid waste products
produced by your body each and every day cannot be adequately
eliminated when the pH of your blood falls into a chronically acidic
state. As your body struggles to restore proper pH balance, excess
wastes start to overwhelm the system. In the process, these waste
products can severely compromise the integrity of your cells and
seriously impair their ability to function properly. In addition, the
waste products prevent the cells from receiving adequate oxygen and
nutrients, and can even disrupt the cells' ability to communicate with
one another.

In Chapter 3, we examined the ways in which your body
attempts to restore pH balance by eliminating and neutralizing
excess acid buildup. If these mechanisms are unable to completely
neutralize accumulated acids, the next step your body takes is to
divert the acids away from vital organs. When this occurs, your body
starts storing the acids in your tissues, joints, and bones. If this
process continues, you are likely to develop joint and skeletal problems such as osteo- and rheumatoid arthritis, and possibly gout. You
may also develop skin conditions, such as dermatitis and eczema;
and/or tissues problems, such as chronic fatigue and fibromyalgia.
Although these conditions can certainly be debilitating, they are not
life-threatening. But if acidosis continues, eventually toxic acids will
start to be stored in vital organs. This can lead to far more serious
health problems, including diabetes, heart disease, and cancer.

To a large degree, the type of disease you develop will depend on
the susceptibility of your individual organs to the effects of toxic
wastes. If, for example, your gastrointestinal tract is most susceptible,
you will be at increased risk for conditions such as colitis, Crohn's
disease, diverticulitis, or stomach cancer. But if the acids, instead, target the myelin sheath, which serves as a protective layer of insulation
around the nerve fibers of the central nervous system, the nerve
impulses that travel from the brain to the muscles can be impaired,
resulting in conditions such as multiple sclerosis. The name of the
disease you develop is not as important as the underlying cause—
toxic buildup of acid wastes due to a chronic state of over-acidity in
your bloodstream.

As acid wastes continue to accumulate, the cells' ability to absorb oxygen and nutrients eventually becomes blocked. This occurs as the cell walls are coated with acidic waste products, losing their permeability. If this process is unchecked, the cell walls then start to harden and solidify. In response, the cells spill out additional waste products in the form of carbon dioxide and lactic acid. This, in turn, increases the acidic environment, dropping pH levels even further.

If this process is not reversed, the cells become covered in extracellular waste and start to die off prematurely. Premature cell death is followed by the decay of the body's tissues and organs. As this occurs, bacteria, fungi, molds, parasites, and other pathogens—all of which thrive in states of acidosis—begin to feed on the diseased areas of the body. As they do, they produce additional waste products that further reduce pH levels, and place an even greater burden on the body.

To better understand this process, picture what happens when a penny is dropped into a vat of acid. Almost immediately, the acid starts to corrode the penny. Eventually, this corrosion completely eats away at the penny, and the acid solution becomes a stagnant, murky chemical swamp. In much the same way, acidosis, left unchecked, corrodes the body from the inside out. In the process, it disrupts and impedes all of the body's internal functions—including immune response, circulation, digestion, hormone production, and neurofunction—leading to various states of disease.

Conventional Medicine's Failure to Address the pH Factor

Doctors all too often ignore the steady decline of the body's organs and their functions resulting from imbalanced pH. I maintain that this is why conventional medicine has so little success reversing chronic disease as opposed to merely managing symptoms. The problem is further compounded by the fact that the very drugs prescribed by conventional physicians to manage chronic disease symptoms actually add to the body's acidic burden.

Most pharmaceutical drugs, especially antibiotics, are acid-producing by nature. Using them to treat health conditions that are primarily caused by over-acidity is like trying to extinguish a fire by lighting matches. Although pharmaceutical drugs absolutely have their place in modern medicine—when used to treat acute, life-threatening disease conditions—their prolonged use for nonacute chronic conditions invariably only serves to make the patients' problems worse. It is therefore no wonder that so many people deveiop complications far beyond their original health complaints. Drugs prescribed to manage the symptoms of these complaints, combined with the state of acidosis that already exists, invariably lead to further deterioration in the body.

If we are to succeed in resolving our nation's growing health crisis, we must look towards a solution that provides us with real answers—answers that can restore and maximize health. As a start, we must understand that most of the major chronic degenerative diseases that face us today are primarily the result of unrecognized stages of acidosis and nutritional deficiencies. Pharmaceutical drugs are certainly capable of relieving pain and suppressing symptoms. But since they are neither alkalizing nor nutritive, they do not address the core problem—they only exacerbate it. And it is unlikely that our medical system will, on its own, radically shift its focus to understanding and treating the real *causes* of disease. Change will arise only when patients demand a different mode of treatment. By understanding the problem of acid-alkaline imbalance and its relationship to health, we can reverse the growing tide of degenerative diseases one person at a time, stemming the health-care crisis we now face.

COMMON DISEASES CAUSED BY ACID-ALKALINE IMBALANCE

It is estimated that between 80 to 85 percent of all disease conditions in the United States are of a chronic, degenerative nature. Such conditions usually do not physically make themselves known until we are in our forties or even later. Given what is known about the relationship between the pH Factor and health, I believe the reason so many of these conditions do not occur earlier in life is that we are born with a healthy acid-alkaline balance that is kept in check by the body's inborn regulatory mechanisms. Because our bodies are designed to heal themselves, it takes many years of bad habits to create a toxic acid buildup powerful enough to disable our healing mechanisms. Only then do chronic health problems become apparent. But the acidic imbalance leading to their manifestation begins much earlier. Based on the relationship between proper pH and good health, let's examine some of the most common disease conditions that are directly related to acid-alkaline imbalance.

ALLERGIES

Allergies are triggered by *allergens*—offending substances found in foods or the environment. Among the most common symptoms of allergies are red, itchy, or watery eyes; sneezing; runny nose; post-nasal drip; swollen sinuses; and skin reactions such as rashes.

Earlier in the book, you learned how a chronically over-acidic environment leads to inflammation. This inflammation causes the body to become hypersensitive to invaders such as dust, pollen, and other allergens. Although a specific allergen may trigger a reaction, it would not occur if the system was not already irritated by its over-acidic state, and therefore highly reactive. Fortunately, by reducing your body's acid load and restoring proper pH balance, allergic reactions can be minimized or eliminated altogether.

In my practice, I've seen this repeatedly borne out by my clients with allergies. Once they start to balance their pH by implementing the nutritional strategies discussed in Chapters 5 and 6, their allergy symptoms become less and less severe or are completely eliminated.

ANXIETY AND DEPRESSION

Although many psychological and social factors can contribute to anxiety and depression, on a biochemical level, both conditions are related to hormonal imbalances. People who are chronically anxious or depressed usually have low levels of serotonin, a hormone that acts as a "feel good" neurotransmitter in the brain. In other cases, although serotonin levels are adequate, the hormone is not properly absorbed by the cells. Although conventional medicine has developed an ever-increasing array of drugs to address the anxiety and depression caused by serotonin deficiencies, such drugs bring with them the risk of serious side effects and, at best, are capable only of controlling symptoms. In and of themselves, they are not complete solutions. A better approach is to understand the relationship between these problems and that of over-acidity.

The condition of over-acidity can interfere with the function of serotonin in two ways. First, it can actually prevent sufficient amounts of the hormone from being produced. Second, it can prevent it from being absorbed by the brain. For the absorption process to function properly, the brain cell membranes must be in a state of semipermeability so that serotonin and other vital nutrients can readily pass through the cell walls. In an acidic state, however, cellular membranes begin to harden, making the absorption process increasingly difficult. So even if enough serotonin is produced, the brain cells can no longer absorb it.

Physicians often prescribe medications called SSRIs (selective serotonin reuptake inhibitors) that literally drive serotonin into the cells. Over time, however, the cells of patients on these medications tend to build up a resistance to the drugs. This makes it necessary for physicians to increase the patient's dose or switch to a different medication.

All of these challenges can usually be avoided by shifting the body's pH levels to a slightly greater alkaline state. Doing so allows the cells to regain their permeability so that serotonin and other hormones, along with nutrients, can once again be readily absorbed.

ARTHRITIS AND GOUT

There are three main types of arthritis: osteoarthritis, rheumatoid arthritis, and gout. One of the primary culprits in each of these arthritic conditions is the excessive buildup of acids in the body. In the case of gout, conventional and alternative physicians agree that uric acid buildup is the cause of the disorder. However, most conventional physicians are unaware of the link between acid buildup and the incidence of osteo- and rheumatoid arthritis.

Osteoarthritis

Osteoarthritis is characterized by the breakdown of cartilage and smooth tissues found at the end of the bones. As the disorder progresses and protective tissue is destroyed, the bones make direct contact with each other, creating friction that causes bone spurs and abnormal bone hardening. The result is severe and potentially debilitating pain.

A common misconception about osteoarthritis is that it is a natural consequence of aging. If that were so, osteoarthritis would be prevalent in all cultures around the world. Among populations whose traditional diets are slightly alkaline, though, osteoarthritis and other forms of arthritis are virtually nonexistent.

The various causative factors that have been linked to osteo-arthritis include free-radical damage, nutritional deficienies, and allergies. As explained in this chapter, all of these factors are related to chronic acidity, and can be eliminated through a diet rich in alka-lizing foods. As this occurs, symptoms of osteoarthritis inevitably resolve themselves as well.

Rheumatoid Arthritis

Rheumatoid arthritis is an inflammatory condition caused by the body's immune system attacking its own healthy tissues. Although this disorder can affect many of the body's organs, it most common-ly causes inflammation of the joints and surrounding tissues. As the disease progresses, the joints become increasingly swollen, painful, and susceptible to deformity.

The most commonly accepted causes of rheumatoid arthritis are food allergies, nutritional deficiencies, internal toxicity, and un-healthy organisms. Again, all of these factors are directly related to excessive acidity. Therefore, unless efforts are focused on reducing stored acids in the body, long-term resolution of rheumatoid arthri-tis is unlikely.

Gout

Every day, uric acid is formed as a byproduct of the body's metabo-lism, and is then eliminated through urination. Proper elimination of uric acid is essential because this substance can neither be destroyed nor stored safely in the body. Unfortunately, because of the modern diet with its excessive consumption of protein-rich foods, our bodies tend to produce excessive amounts of uric acid—far more than the body can handle.

As excess uric acid finds its way into the bloodstream, it can trav-el to any part of the body. As it does so, it becomes solidified as uric acid crystals, which are then deposited in tissues and joints. Over time, this accumulated buildup of uric acid begins to destroy carti-lage and to irritate the joints, causing the swelling and severe pain associated with gout.

Modern medicine primarily treats gout—as well as other forms of arthritis—with anti-inflammatory and pain-relief medicines. As we have discussed, however, such measures often serve to aggravate the problem due to the acidifying effect of such drugs. When patients choose instead to start eating primarily alkalizing foods, the body is able to eliminate the stored uric acid crystals, and the symptoms of gout are eliminated as well.

CANCER

In 1931, German biochemist Dr. Otto Warburg was awarded the Nobel Prize for conclusively showing that cancer arises and spreads in the body due to a lack of oxygen. "All normal cells have an absolute requirement for oxygen, but cancer cells can live without oxygen—a rule *without any exception*," he wrote. As part of his research, Dr. Warburg took healthy, normal cells from an embryo and forced them to grow in a petri dish without oxygen. He found that the cells would soon take on all the characteristics of cancer cells due to oxygen deprivation. His experiment revealed that all normal, healthy cells in the body may be transformed into cancer cells if they are unable to obtain sufficient oxygen.

Further research by Dr. Warburg showed that when cells are oxygen-deprived, they regress into a "primitive state" and start obtaining energy from the fermentation of glucose, a form of sugar. Healthy cells, by contrast, derive their energy from oxygen. Moreover, the fermentation process can occur only in the absence of oxygen at the cellular level. Cells that subsist on glucose fermentation burden the body by producing large amounts of lactic acid, a waste product that further increases acidity, making it even more difficult for healthy cells to obtain and make use of oxygen. This leads to the further spread of cancerous cells, which, if left unchecked, clump together to form tumors. According to Drs. W. John Diamond and W. Lee Cowden, authors of *An Alternative Medicine Definitive Guide to Cancer*, research has shown that cancerous cells can contain as much as ten times more lactic acid than healthy cells.

This proven link between cancer, oxygen deprivation, and pH levels is almost completely ignored in this country, according to Drs. Diamond and Cowden. They write, "Most of the physicians trained in the United States fail to realize that blood pH balance is critical in determining whether or not tumor [cancer] cells thrive or die." By contrast, nonconventional physicians who are having success in treating cancer pay close attention to their patients' blood pH levels, doing everything they can to shift pH levels back to a healthy acid-alkaline balance that allows for appropriate oxygen levels.

It would be irresponsible to say that appropriate adjustment of body pH levels is adequate to prevent and reverse cancer. Numerous factors are involved in the onset of cancer, and all of them must be addressed if long-term remission is to be achieved. As part of the puzzle, though, it makes sense to keep pH levels slightly alkaline, and thereby ensure that the body's cells and tissues are receiving adequate supplies of oxygen.

CARDIOVASCULAR DISEASE

Your body's cardiovascular system is an interconnected highway of arteries, veins, and capillaries, at the center of which lies the heart. It is the heart that acts as a pump which drives blood—along with the oxygen, nutrients, and other essential elements it contains—throughout the rest of the cardiovascular system, feeding your cells and organs. It is also the heart that regulates blood pressure and circulation. The entire cardiovascular system is designed to operate in a slightly alkaline environment.

When blood pH becomes acidic, the acids in the blood act like chemical irritants, eroding the cell wall membranes of the heart, arteries, veins, and cardiovascular connective tissues. Acid buildup also interferes with the ability of the heart and arteries to properly contract and relax as blood is pumped through the cardiovascular system. In addition, excess acids elevate cholesterol levels, which then solidify and are deposited in the blood vessels, leading to plaque buildup. All of these factors contribute to arteriosclerosis (hardening of the arteries), aneurysm (widening and ballooning of artery walls), arrhythmia (abnormal heartbeat), heart attack, hypertension (high blood pressure), and stroke.

Acidosis also affects the cardiovascular system by allowing infectious organisms to thrive in the bloodstream. Researchers in Italy have found that an estimated 85 percent of all patients suffering from cardiovascular disease also have concentrations of cytomegalovirus (CMV) in their heart tissue. CMV places a further strain on the heart, but the virus's ability to thrive is significantly reduced when blood pH returns to a slightly alkaline state. This can be accomplished by eating primarily alkalizing foods.

DIABETES

An overly acidic pH is directly related to what is known as adult-onset diabetes, or Type II diabetes. Type II diabetes accounts for the majority of diabetes cases, and is increasing in epidemic proportions in the United States. The most common trait among populations suffering from Type II diabetes is a diet high in acid-producing foods.

Type II diabetes occurs when the body becomes overly acidic, causing body tissues to resist the attempts of the hormone insulin to deliver glucose to the cells. The body, which uses insulin to regulate glucose and maintain proper blood sugar levels, then produces excessive amounts of insulin. In order to cope with this excess insulin, the body produces more fat in which to store it. It is for this reason that people with Type II diabetes are so often overweight. It is commonly thought that being overweight triggers Type II diabetes, but it is more accurate to say that both conditions are related to the same underlying cause—acidosis.

This problem is further compounded by the effect of the body's acidic environment on the pancreas's beta cells, which are responsible for producing and secreting insulin. The beta cells are highly sensitive to pH levels, and when bathed in acids, are unable to properly function and survive. Forced to produce insulin under increasingly worsening conditions, the cells become less effective at communicating with one another. In addition, acidic wastes start to accumulate and coat the beta cells, making it more difficult for the cells to produce insulin and for the insulin itself to be properly utilized.

The solution to this problem is to shift the pH to its proper balance. Once the body's internal environment returns to a slightly alkaline state, the symptoms of Type II diabetes start to abate, and in most cases, the condition is eliminated altogether. Interestingly, prior to the use of synthetic insulin shots to treat diabetes, physicians traditionally treated the condition with alkalizing powders.

FATIGUE

Persistent fatigue is usually a sign that your body is laboring in a state of chronic acidosis. An acidic pH both drains the body's production of energy and interferes with its ability to make use of its energy reserves. The result is a lack of vitality.

To better understand how acidosis impairs the body's production and utilization of energy, you need to understand how energy is created in the body at the cellular level. Under normal, healthy conditions, the cells' own internal energy factories, the mitochondria, produce energy using a fuel called adenosine triphosphate (ATP), a substance synthesized from oxygen and glucose. ATP, in turn, is essential for powering the cells' sodium-potassium pumps. The primary role of the sodium-potassium pumps is to maintain the proper balance between sodium and potassium within and without the cell walls. Inside the cells, the potassium has to remain high and the sodium has to remain low for the body's energy, which is electrical in nature, to be generated. Outside the cell, the concentrations of sodium and potassium are reversed—potassium levels are low, and sodium levels are high. According to Dr. Samuel West, ND, founder of the International Academy of Lymphology, "Because the potassium is high within the cell and low outside it, it automatically seeps outside the cell. It will go from high concentration to low concentration. And the sodium does the same, except it seeps into the cell. If this seepage is not reversed by the sodium-potassium pumps, you get disease or death. The pumps are what keep this delicate balance intact, and to work they require the energy supplied them by the mitochondria via the ATP."

Acidosis interferes with this process by diminishing the supply of oxygen to the cells. With less oxygen available to interact with glucose, less ATP can be produced. This, in turn, causes less energy to be available throughout the body.

Another factor associated with low energy levels is diminished enzyme activity. As explained in Chapter 3, enzymes act as catalysts for every chemical reaction that occurs in the body, including those used in the production and utilization of energy, and proper pH is essential for optimal enzyme function. When pH levels become imbalanced, the ability of enzymes to perform their tasks is impaired and, in an acidic state, enzymes can be deactivated altogether.

The solution to chronic fatigue, therefore, lies in restoring the body's available oxygen supply and ensuring that enzymatic reactions take place in a suitable internal environment. Both of these goals can be accomplished in large part by restoring the body's proper pH balance.

GASTROINTESTINAL DISORDERS

As we saw in Chapter 3, most gastrointestinal (GI) disorders are caused by an acid-alkaline imbalance. These problems include acid reflux, colitis, constipation, Crohn's disease, diarrhea, diverticulitis, dyspepsia, flatulence, indigestion, and irritable bowel syndrome (IBS).

In an overly acidic state, the body's digestive enzymes are unable to adequately perform their functions. To compensate for diminished enzyme activity, the body secretes more acids, which can lead to indigestion. Additionally, as enzyme function continues to be impaired, the foods that pass through the GI tract are only partially digested, and therefore cannot supply the body with all of the nutrients it needs. This, in turn, leads to fermentation of the undigested food particles, creating waste products that accumulate in the GI tract. These waste products adhere to the intestinal walls and further hamper the absorption of vital nutrients, causing inflammatory conditions such as colitis, Crohn's disease, and diverticulitis.

Before long, this buildup of waste products begins to interfere with proper bowel function, meaning that toxins which would normally be eliminated from the body are not. Instead, they too start to accumulate in the body. The result is a state of chronic toxicity in the GI tract that eventually spreads to other areas of the body. It is for this reason that many holistic physicians say, "Death begins in the colon."

These gastrointestinal problems can all be prevented and reversed by a diet that primarily includes alkalizing foods. All of my clients who suffer from GI disorders show substantial improvement once they eliminate acid-forming foods from their diet and replace them with alkali-forming foods. As this occurs, enzyme activity in the body once again builds to normal levels. Where appropriate, this process can be helped by supplementation with digestive enzymes. (See Chapter 6 for more information about supplementation.)

KIDNEY DISEASE

When blood pH remains acidic, acid waste products accumulate over time in the bloodstream. The kidneys, which serve as the filtration system for the blood, then become overburdened. Eventually, if acid waste increases to the point where the kidneys cannot filter it out, a variety of kidney conditions can occur, including nephritis (kidney inflammation), uremia (excess waste products in the blood), and the formation of bladder and/or kidney stones.

Contrary to popular belief, bladder and kidney stones are composed of crystals of uric acid, phosphoric acid, and/or oxalic acid—not excess calcium. Calcium compounds dissolve in urine that is acidic, while bladder and kidney stones do not. Whether the problem is kidney stones or another kidney-related problem, the two main keys to avoiding and reversing such disorders are to drink adequate amounts of water throughout the day, and to move away from a diet that is acid-producing. Eating primarily alkali-producing foods to regain a proper pH balance can prevent such conditions altogether. If the problems already exist, these steps can eliminate the disorder. In the case of kidney or bladder stones, for instance, over time they will dissolve by themselves once the internal environment becomes slightly alkaline, and can then be flushed out of the body by drinking water. As discussed in Chapter 2, a general rule of thumb for adequate daily water intake is to drink half an ounce of water for every pound of body weight, e.g., 75 ounces—or about 9 cups—for a person weighing 150 pounds.

OSTEOPOROSIS

When pH levels remain chronically acidic, the body is forced to leech calcium supplies from the bones and teeth in an attempt to neutralize the acids. This process places stress on both bones and teeth, and is a primary cause of osteoporosis, a disease in which bones become thin and porous.

Osteoporosis is the most prevalent form of bone disorder in the United States, with an estimated 10 million Americans suffering from this condition, and another 18 million at high risk. Additionally, 1.5 million bone fractures occur each year in this country due to osteoporosis, primarily within the spine, hips, or wrists.

In her book *Better Bones, Better Body*, Susan Brown, PhD, a world-renowned medical anthropologist and clinical nutritionist, writes: "[O]steoporosis is a common condition with serious consequences for one third of older females and perhaps 15 to 20 percent of all older males in this country." Dr. Brown also states that osteoporosis is a "needless disorder" and "a disease of Western civilization created by our lifestyles." By contrast, she points out that osteoporosis is "unknown or uncommon among indigenous and traditional peoples living their time-honored lifestyles."

The reason osteoporosis is so rare among indigenous peoples that their traditional diets are highly alkalizing in nature. While this fact has long been proven and accepted by Dr. Brown and her fellow anthropologists, it seems to be completely ignored by the Western medical community, which chooses instead to manage osteoporosis with synthetic hormone therapy and drugs designed to increase bone density. Such approaches, while capable of providing symptomatic relief, do not usually solve the problem. Far greater success rates have been achieved by Dr. Brown's Better Bones, Better Body Program™, a self-care approach based on the doctor's research findings. One centerpiece of this program is a diet rich in alkalizing foods. I employ this same dietary approach in my clinical practice, and am happy to report that those clients who commit to the program inevitably experience a resolution of their osteoporosis symptoms. Once again, the key lies in restoring proper pH balance.

PREMATURE AGING AND RELATED CONDITIONS

Scientists have long linked premature aging with free-radical damage. A free radical is an unstable molecule. As it collides with other molecules, its overall effect is to break down cells and cell membranes; harmfully alter proteins, enzymes, fatty acids, hormones, and even DNA; and diminish the ability of the body's organs and systems to effectively do their jobs. Because an overly acidic environment increases free-radical production, people who suffer from acidosis are far more likely to suffer from premature aging than those who maintain balanced pH levels. As long as the body's internal environment remains acidic, free radicals flourish, continuing their rampage of cellular destruction. This results in a number of problems, including wrinkled, sagging skin, age spots, and other signs of aging. Free radicals can also damage mitochondria, the cell's energy factories, resulting in greater fatigue and an overall reduction in organ function.

As explained in Chapter 3, acidosis can also contribute to premature aging by inhibiting neuron activity, and thereby impairing brain function. This can result in forgetfulness, confusion, and disorientation. The lack of oxygen and nutrients associated with acidosis further compounds the problem.

As you might expect, premature aging can, for the most part, be avoided and to some degree reversed by the adoption of a diet rich in alkalizing foods. Such a diet prevents free-radical damage, enables neurons to function properly, and provides the brain with the oxygen and nutrients it needs.

RESPIRATORY CONDITIONS

There are three general categories of respiratory conditions: infections such as the common cold, pneumonia, sinusitis, and tuberculosis; chronic lung diseases such as asthma and bronchitis; and respiratory conditions caused by chemical/environmental agents such as asbestos, dust, pollen, and so forth. Your susceptibility to conditions in all three categories is directly related to the acidity of your blood. As we discussed in Chapter 3, respiration is one of the ways that the body regulates acid-alkaline balance, chiefly by removing carbon dioxide and acids from the blood. When the body's internal environment is in a state of chronic acidosis, however, this regulatory process is disrupted. As a result, higher levels of carbon dioxide and acids remain in the bloodstream, leaving less oxygen available for the cells and tissues.

We have already discussed how this acidic environment is an ideal breeding ground for bacteria, viruses, fungi, and parasites. All of these pathogens can cause respiratory problems. Moreover, research has now confirmed that certain viruses—such as coronaviruses and rhinoviruses, which are the primary cause of the common cold, and influenza viruses—can infect the body's cells only by attaching themselves to cellular membranes when the body is in an acidic state. For this reason, such viruses are called pH-dependent.

Strains of the coronavirus are particularly dependent on acidity. For example, research has shown that the MHV-A59 coronavirus thrives in a pH of 6.0, but rapidly weakens and dies when pH levels are briefly raised to 8.0. As another example, the murine coronavirus A59 has been shown to be ten times more infectious in a pH of 6.0, compared with a pH of 7.0.

According to the tenets of acupuncture and traditional Chinese medicine (TCM), respiratory conditions are also associated with the health of the colon and gastrointestinal tract. When the GI tract is overly acidic, pathogens thrive and migrate throughout the rest of the body, often settling within the upper chest and lungs, and leading to conditions such as chronic bronchitis and pneumonia. For this reason, TCM practitioners usually seek to cleanse and detoxify the GI tract when treating respiratory conditions. From my own clinical experience, I find that both measures are most effectively accomplished by placing patients on an alkalizing diet. As their pH shifts from overly acidic to slightly alkaline, symptoms invariably disappear and overall health improves.

SKIN CONDITIONS

Surface skin cells are replaced every thirty days. Ideally, when skin cells regenerate, they are healthy and vibrant, but for most people this is not the case. What keeps healthy regeneration from occurring—not only for skin cells, but for all the cells, tissues, and organs of the body—is over-acidity and associated toxins. Perspiration is one of the ways in which the body regulates acid-alkaline balance. But toxic buildup caused by over-acidity can clog skin pores, resulting in a variety of skin conditions, including eczema and psoriasis. Then such problems are exacerbated as the liver attempts to cleanse and detoxify itself while coping with the burdens of acidosis. Overall, the problems posed by acidity create a vicious cycle that can wreak havoc on individuals predisposed to skin conditions.

Over the years, many clients have come to me suffering from eczema and psoriasis, as well as other skin conditions. Often eczema and psoriasis go hand in hand, and have afflicted these individuals for many years. But in every single case, these conditions are significantly relieved when clients adopt a diet of alkalizing foods and plentiful amounts of pure water.

VISION PROBLEMS

Vision problems can also occur as a result of acidosis—a possibility generally not considered by physicians and optometrists. As excessive acidity causes oxygen levels to diminish within the cells, glucose stores that would normally combine with oxygen to fuel the mitochondria instead bind with protein molecules, causing the cells of the eye to harden and lose their flexibility. In addition, calcium deposits formed as a result of acidosis can accumulate on the optic nerves. When this occurs, the result can be cataracts, macular degeneration, and vision loss.

WEIGHT GAIN AND OBESITY

Although recent research indicates that some people have a genetic predisposition to excessive weight gain, genes are not the sole determinant of health. The choices we make about our health are just as important. When we choose our lifestyles and eating habits wisely, good health—including ideal weight levels and abundant energy—is attainable.

Unfortunately, in the United States, the choices being made are increasingly unhealthy ones. A lack of physical exercise, a high-stress lifestyle, and poor dietary choices are combining to create a state of chronic acidosis. As a result, obesity is becoming a problem of epidemic proportions.

How does acidosis lead to obesity? When pH levels become and remain acidic, the body produces fat cells to encapsulate and transport excess acids away from the organs. This is done to safeguard the organs from the damage that the acids would otherwise cause. But if this process is carried out on a long-term basis, unhealthy weight gain is the inevitable result.

Moreover, the ability to digest and assimilate nutrients from any foods consumed—even healthy foods—starts to diminish as acidity continues, and the yeasts that thrive in an acidic environment start to interfere with the digestive process. As the liver strives to cope with the buildup of acidic toxins, its ability to efficiently metabolize fats and sugars also diminishes. Both of these factors compound the problems of weight gain and obesity, resulting in nutritional deficiencies that leave you feeling hungry even after you have eaten. Thus a vicious cycle is set in motion in which the body, through hunger pangs, attempts to receive the nutrients it requires.

Another consequence of acidosis that contributes to excessive weight gain is hormonal imbalance, which can affect the adrenal and thyroid glands. As hormonal function is thrown off by over-acidity, the adrenal glands have to work overtime, eventually to the point of exhaustion. This leads to lower energy levels, making it difficult to engage in exercise and other physical activities that burn calories. At the same time, the thyroid, which helps regulate metabolism, is negatively impacted, leading to cravings for sugar and other unhealthy foods as the body seeks desperately to supply itself with energy.

Dire as the above picture seems, I have repeatedly seen obese and overweight people dramatically and permanently shed excess pounds once they began eating alkalizing foods. Just as important, my clients have done so safely, instead of following unwise diets— diets that can artificially inhibit appetite, placing a strain on the body and leading to the so-called "yo-yo effect," in which weight is regained once the diet is over. As pH levels return to normal, the body once again becomes able to obtain the nutrients it needs without signaling the desire to overeat. Energy reserves then increase, and the individual is once again able to pursue a regular routine of exercise and physical activity.

CONCLUSION

This chapter has shown the dangers posed to your health by acid-alkaline imbalances. I've chosen to focus on the most common conditions that can result from chronic pH imbalance, but based on my clinical experience, I would have to say that nearly every disease is related to this factor. For that reason, I maintain that it is far more important to correct the imbalances that cause the disease than to focus on the specific disease itself. The condition that ultimately manifests itself depends on the system or systems within your body that are weakest and most susceptible to their attack.

Were the public and their physicians more aware of this principle, I believe that we as a nation would soon become much healthier. But you do not have to wait for a shift in public awareness to improve your health. The tools you need to achieve and maintain acid-alkaline balance are available right now, starting with proper diet. This is the subject we will explore in the next chapter.

5

Getting Back
in Balance

pproximately 2,500 years ago, Hippocrates, the father of Western medicine, advised, "Let food be thy medicine and let medicine be thy food." Since that time, this has been a basic tenet of holistic physicians. It is also fundamental to achieving and maintaining proper pH, for it is primarily the foods you eat that influence the acid-alkaline balance of your body's internal environment.

Most American diets are high in foods that lead to imbalanced pH levels, as evidenced by the soaring incidence of chronic diseases facing our nation. This chapter focuses on shifting that trend by eating wisely. By incorporating the following guidelines into your daily life, you will soon find yourself experiencing renewed health and greater energy.

HOW THE FOODS YOU EAT
AFFECT YOUR BODY'S ACID-ALKALINE BALANCE

Once they are digested and metabolized—literally burned down—all foods leave a residue of ash in your body. Depending on the type of food and its mineral content, the ash residue is either acidic or alkaline. Foods that produce an acidic ash have an acidifying effect on the body, and therefore lower pH levels. Foods that leave an alkaline ash have the effect of raising pH levels. Generally speaking, foods eaten raw tend to have an alkalizing effect on pH levels, compared with cooked foods, which typically are acidifying in nature.

It is important to note that the acidifying or alkalizing effects of the foods you eat are far more significant, in terms of your health, than the foods' inherent pH values prior to their consumption. For example, a number of foods that are acidic in nature, such as certain citrus fruits and vinegars, actually have a strongly alkalizing effect on the body after they are digested and metabolized. Not all acidic foods are acidifying when they are eaten, nor are all alkaline foods alkalizing when consumed. Therefore, the key to choosing your foods wisely is to fully understand the effect that each food will have on your body's pH levels.

Ironically, the acidifying and alkalizing effects of foods are too often ignored by dieticians and nutritionists, who focus solely on the foods' nutrient content. Nutrients are, of course, essential to good health. But as Chapter 4 explained, when pH levels are imbalanced, proper absorption and utilization of nutrients is interrupted, eventually resulting in nutritional deficiencies. Fortunately, by following the guidelines presented in this chapter, you will be able to achieve optimal pH levels and obtain all the nutrients your body needs.

BASIC GUIDELINES

Before you learn which foods are acidifying and which are alkalizing, it's important to become familiar with a handful of guidelines that can help you make better food selections. In general, alkalizing foods should constitute between 60 and 80 percent of your diet. If your pH levels are more than slightly acidic, alkalizing foods should compose approximately 80 percent of your daily dietary intake. The basic rule of thumb is this: The more you suffer from over-acidity, the more alkalizing foods you should consume.

It is also important to eat alkalizing foods at *every* meal, rather than eating all your alkalizing foods at one or two meals and eating acidifying foods the rest of the day. This absolutely includes snacks. And never try to eat meals that consist solely of acidifying foods, such as pasta with meatballs.

When you eat a higher proportion of alkalizing foods at every meal, your body becomes better able to neutralize whatever acids are produced during digestion, so eating this way will safeguard your body from the burden of further acidity. It will also allow your body's detoxification system to more effectively reduce and eliminate those toxic acids that have already built up inside of you.

If you are like most people, in order to improve you health, you may need to eat greater amounts of alkalizing foods initially. But over time, as your pH levels become more balanced, you will be able to lower the percentage of alkalizing foods and still maintain good health. Once you achieve and stabilize your ideal pH level, you may even find that you can eat equal amounts of alkalizing and acidifying foods without any problems. Overall, however, I recommend that you continue to eat a higher proportion of alkalizing foods even after your health and energy levels have returned to normal.

Since alkalizing foods play a significant role in bringing overly acidic pH levels into balance, you may think it wise to drastically reduce your intake of acidifying foods, or to eliminate them altogether. *Don't!* No matter how acidic your pH may be, your body still requires foods that are rich in proteins in order to function properly. Foods with the highest concentration of proteins are meat, fish, eggs, and dairy products, all of which have highly acidifying effects on the body. But if you eliminate such foods from your diet altogether, you will not be able to achieve acid-alkaline balance.

The body requires a certain amount of acidifying protein in order to establish alkaline minerals in the tissues. It is protein that enables your tissues to retain these vital alkaline minerals. By eliminating all protein, you will eliminate some of those minerals that protect you when harmful acids need to be neutralized. When this occurs, the acids spread throughout your body, forcing it to call on stored mineral reserves, eventually to the point where those reserves are completely depleted. The result is greater acidity and the possible onset of disease.

There may be times when an all-alkaline diet is warranted, such as in cases of pronounced acidosis accompanied by painful symptoms. But an all-alkaline diet should be followed only for a short period of time—no more than one or two weeks. By following an entirely alkaline diet of vegetables and fruits, the body will have a chance to recover more rapidly. But because of the lack of protein, it would not be wise to continue on such a diet once symptoms have abated.

Of course, the above guidelines should *not* be followed by people whose pH levels are overly alkaline. Admittedly, such people are rare, given the highly acidifying effects of the standard American diet, but if you fall into this category, you will want to increase your intake of acidifying foods until your pH returns to normal. After that, you will want to monitor your pH and follow the guidelines above. (See Table 5.1 for more specific dietary guidelines.)

TABLE 5.1. PH EATING PLANS		
pH Level	Recommended Percentage of Acidifying Foods in Diet	Recommended Percentage of Alkalizing Foods in Diet
Too Alkaline	40% to 50%	50% to 60%
Normal	20% to 40%	60% to 80%
Too Acidic	20%	80%
Extremely Acidic*	0%	100%

*The diet of 100% alkalizing foods should be followed for one to two weeks only, after which the "Too Acidic" diet should be followed.

ACIDIFYING AND ALKALIZING FOODS

As we've discussed, the foods we eat can be divided into two distinct categories in terms of their effect on pH levels: acidifying or alkalizing. However, it is also important to know the degree to which foods produce their effects. For example, grains such as brown rice and millet both have an acidifying effect on the body, but brown rice is far less acidifying than millet.

Compounding this issue is the fact that your unique biochemistry has its own inherent strengths and weakness with regard to how the foods you eat affect you. As you begin to adopt the specific eating plan I am recommending, you will want to pay careful attention to how you feel following each meal. A food that produces only a mildly acidifying effect for most people might be very acidifying for you. Should this occur, trust your experience and modify your food selections accordingly. In general, however, the information presented in this chapter—which specifies whether foods are acidifying or alkalizing—is accurate for the vast majority of people.

Acidifying Foods

Acidifying foods are generally high in proteins, carbohydrates, and/or fats. Such foods include:

Alcohol

Breads

Caffeine products (chocolate, coffee, black tea)

Milk and other dairy products

Poultry

Refined and processed foods

Commercial condiments	Seeds and nuts
Fish	Soda
Certain grains	Sugar and artificial sweeteners
Legumes	Tap water
Meats	Yeast products

Alcohol. All alcoholic beverages cause acidification in the body. In addition, excessive alcohol consumption has been linked to a number of serious disorders, most especially alcoholism and cirrhosis of the liver.

While recent research indicates that moderate consumption of beer or wine can enhance health by relieving stress and improving digestion, I recommend that when you drink alcohol, you limit yourself to a glass of beer or wine, and you accompany it with a glass of water to minimize the alcohol's acidifying effects.

Breads. All breads are acidifying. Some, however, are more so than others. Whole-grain breads are less acidifying than breads made with refined grains, for instance, and yeast-free breads are less acidifying than yeast breads. As a rule, eat bread sparingly, if at all, and avoid white breads and yeast breads entirely. If you do choose to eat bread, toast it first to neutralize its acidifying effects.

Caffeine Products. Foods in this group include chocolate, cocoa, teas, and all forms of coffee, including decaffeinated coffees. Caffeine produces high amounts of acidic residues in the body, and is also mucus-forming. According to Drs. Robert S. Ivker and Robert A. Anderson, over 50 percent of all Americans are addicted to caffeine, primarily in the form of coffee, which they consume throughout the day for the burst of energy it provides. Ironically, caffeine actually drains the body's energy reserves, creating a harmful cycle in which the caffeine drinker need another cup of coffee as soon as the artificial energy jolt from the last cup wears off.

Condiments. The primary offenders in this category are mayonnaise, ketchup, and mustard, all prized staples of the standard American diet. Why are these products harmful? Most commercial condiments contain sugar as well as other unhealthy additives. If you don't wish to eliminate these products completely, at least use them sparingly and choose brands that are organic. Better yet, consider using healthy substitutes such as natural herbs and spices, sea salt, or kelp to add flavor to the dishes you prepare.

Fish, Meat, and Poultry. All meats and meat byproducts—including not only beef and pork, but also fish and poultry—have an acidifying effect on the body because of their high protein content. After such foods are digested and metabolized, they leave behind residues of uric acid, which can cause toxic acid buildup in the body. Meats also contain phosphorus and sulfur, two minerals that also are acidifying. In addition, commercially harvested meats, fish, and poultry are usually laced with hormones, pesticides, steroids, and antibiotics, all of which are harmful to your health.

Animal fats—often used in cooking and deep-frying, and present in all meat, fish, and poultry—contribute to acidic pH because they are high in saturated fatty acids. These fats are difficult for the body to properly digest and metabolize. Incomplete digestion of saturated fatty acids results in the creation of toxic waste products that place a further burden on the body's ability to maintain balanced acid-alkaline levels. Given the high fat content of the standard American diet, it is little wonder that acidification due to unhealthy fat consumption is quite common in the United States.

Grains. Both whole and refined grains—including rice, oats, wheat, and millet—are for the most part acidifying. Grains are primarily composed of carbohydrates, which are often poorly digested due to the fact that many people unknowingly are sensitive or allergic to them. Interestingly, however, when grains are sprouted, they become alkalizing foods, and have positive effects similar to those of green vegetables. For this reason, I recommend that you consider making sprouted grain products a staple of your diet, while using non-sprouted grains sparingly. (See the inset on page 89 to learn more about sprouts.)

Legumes. Legumes are a class of vegetables consisting of beans and peas, as well as some plants commonly thought of as nuts. Included in this group are aduki beans, black beans, black-eyed peas, chick-peas, great northern beans, green beans, green peas, kidney beans, lentils, lima beans, mung beans, navy beans, peanuts, pinto beans, and soybeans. Legumes are low in calories and provide a nice balance of proteins and complex carbohydrates. They are also a staple food for many people around the world.

Unfortunately, legumes create acidic conditions in the body, primarily by leaving a residue of uric acid when they are metabolized. The most acidifying foods in this category are peanuts, chickpeas, and soybeans. Peanut products, such as peanut butter, also fall into this category.

Because legumes are so rich in nutrients, I do not recommend that you eliminate them from your diet. Rather, feel free to include them in your meal plans, but do so in moderation. To further enhance the nutritious benefits they provide, consider sprouting them. (See page 89.) Sprouting not only dramatically reduces legumes' acidifying effects, but also increases their nutritive value.

Milk and Dairy Products. Included in this group are eggs, milk, cheese, and other products made with milk. Be aware that cheeses with a sharp flavor, such as Cheddar, are more acidifying than milder white cheeses. Also keep in mind that in addition to causing acidification, milk and dairy products contain the protein casein, which produces mucus buildup.

Many people are also unknowingly sensitive to milk and dairy products due to their inability to tolerate lactose, also known as milk sugar. Unfortunately, commercial milk also contains a multitude of chemicals that have been found to be unhealthy to humans. These chemicals include hormones, antibiotics, pesticides, and many other substances that are given to cows to increase milk production.

Refined and Processed Foods. The foods found in this category include fast foods; candies; donuts and pastries; refined flours and breads; refined grain products, including white flour pastas; and commercial cereals. These foods are not only highly acidifying, but have also been stripped of essential nutrients through the refinement process. In addition, they contain artificial chemical flavorings, colorings, and preservatives—substances that are completely foreign to the body's digestive system. They are also high in sugars and hydrogenated or partially hydrogenated oils, both of which have been linked to a range of degenerative diseases, including cancer.

Regular consumption of such foods is a sure recipe for major health problems. They should be eliminated completely from your diet.

Seeds and Nuts. With the exception of almonds and Brazil nuts (see page 87 for more information on these nuts), all seeds and nuts lower pH values in the body, creating acidity. Foods in this category include pumpkin, sesame, and sunflower seeds, as well as cashews, hazelnuts, pecans, and walnuts. All of these foods contain phosphorous and sulfur, and are high in fat, all of which can contribute to acidification.

Since seeds and nuts are rich in other nutrients, I am in favor of making them part of your regular food intake, so long as they are eaten in moderation. By soaking seeds and nuts overnight, you can help minimize their acidic effect.

Soda. Soda is one of the most highly acidifying substances you can consume. Not only does soda have a high sugar content, but it often contains high levels of caffeine, further adding to the problem.

To give you a better idea of how toxic the effects of soda are on your body, consider this finding from researcher Sang Wang, author of the book *Reverse Aging*. In order to neutralize one glass of soda, you must drink thirty-two glasses of highly alkaline water. I recommend that you eliminate soda altogether. As a substitute, you may use unflavored seltzer water or club soda, but I suggest that you do so sparingly.

Sugar. According to Drs. Robert Ivker and Robert Anderson, authors of *The Complete Self-Care Guide to Holistic Medicine*, the average American eats 150 pounds of sugar each and every year. This is not all that surprising, since sugar is seemingly everywhere in the standard American diet. It can be found under the following names: white sugar, brown sugar, cane sugar, corn sugar, date sugar, fructose, galactose, glucose, lactose, maltose, mannitol, and sorbitol. Honey, maple syrup, and molasses are other sugar-rich foods.

Commercial white sugar—a staple of jellies, candies, pastries, etc.—is also a refined food, meaning that it contains no vitamins, minerals, or enzymes. The absence of such nutrients makes it extremely difficult for the body to metabolize sugar, forcing it to release stored vitamins and minerals in an attempt to convert sugar to energy. This, in turns, reduces the available supply of stored nutrients that the body would otherwise use to function properly and maintain balanced pH levels.

Sugar poses other serious health risks as well. It is one of the primary substances used by cancer cells to fuel their growth and proliferation, and acts as fuel for numerous harmful microorganisms. As these microorganisms die and decompose, the fermentation they cause increases the body's acidity, creating additional health burdens. For all of these reasons, I recommend that you completely eliminate added sugars from your diet. Foods containing naturally-occurring sugars, especially fruits, are permissible, but should be eaten sparingly, with the exception of avocados, bananas, grapefruit, lemons, and limes, which have alkalizing effects.

Artificial Sweeteners. Many people who seek to eliminate sugar from their diet choose to use artificial sweeteners as substitutes under the mistaken belief that they are healthier. Nothing could be further from the truth. Products such as aspartame (Nutrasweet), saccharine, and cyclamates are extremely acidifying. In addition, a number of the chemical ingredients they contain have been linked to a wide range of disease conditions and symptoms. If you are seeking a healthy substitute for sugar, I recommend stevia or xylitol.

Tap Water. Tap water is not only acidifying, but usually also contains fluoride and chlorine—substances that have been linked to a number of degenerative diseases, including cancer. For this reason, I recommend avoiding tap water altogether, even when steaming vegetables or boiling pasta. Because adequate water intake is so important to your health, consider using water filters or buying bottled alkaline mineral water. (See page 86.)

Yeast Products. Besides brewer's and baker's yeast, this category includes breads and baked goods, beer, and wine. Yeast is also often an ingredient in commercial condiments and seasonings.

Yeast consumption can promote the proliferation of *Candida albicans*, the microorganism responsible for candidiasis, or systemic yeast overgrowth in the body. Candidiasis is a widespread problem among many people suffering from chronic health problems such as allergies, anxiety and depression, chronic fatigue, fungal infections, gastrointestinal disorders, memory problems, mood swings, respiratory problems, and sleep disturbances.

Aside from those products that should be completely eliminated, the foods discussed above can remain part of your diet. You should, however, eat them sparingly, limiting their combined intake to no more than 40 percent of the foods you eat each day, and ideally reducing them to 20 percent of your diet, especially if you are already suffering from chronic health problems. And always remember to eat a greater amount of alkalizing foods at every meal to help neutralize the effects of those acidifying foods you choose to include.

Alkalizing Foods

Alkalizing foods are rich in alkaline minerals and contain little or no acidic substances. In addition, these foods produce no acidic ash when they are digested and metabolized, regardless of the amount consumed at any meal. Foods in this category include:

Alkaline mineral water   Certain nuts

Certain fruits   Sprouts

Cold-pressed oils   Vegetables

Herbs, spices, and salts

Alkaline Mineral Water. Water in its natural state usually has a neutral pH of 7.0. Due to chlorination and fluoridation, however, most tap water has an acidic pH. The same is true of carbonated water. Many brands of mineral water, on the other hand, are alkalizing because of the alkaline minerals they contain. Such brands list their pH values right on the label, making it easy for you to determine their degree of alkalinity.

Fruits. Although fruits are rich in essential nutrients, enzymes, and fiber, they are also abundant in natural sugars. This makes most fruits slightly acidifying. For this reason, most people should eat fruits sparingly.

The exceptions to this rule are bananas, grapefruit, lemons, limes, avocados, and tomatoes. (Although avocados and tomatoes are often considered vegetables, in actuality, they are fruits.) Bananas are naturally alkaline, whereas grapefruit, lemons, and limes are acidic in nature. However, during the digestive process, as grapefruit, lemons, and limes are metabolized, they have a highly alkalizing effect. All three of these citrus fruits are also naturally rich in oxygen, which enhances their alkalizing abilities. As an easy and effective aid in helping your body maintain proper acid-alkaline balance, I recommend beginning each day with a glass of purified water combined with fresh-squeezed lemon juice. Or, if you prefer, you can substitute lime. (Make sure you use organic fruits whenever possible.) This makes an excellent tonic to get your morning started, and is highly alkalizing. To gain full benefits, wait for twenty to thirty minutes before you eat anything.

Although most dried fruits are slightly acidifying, some—apricots, bananas, dates, and raisins—are mildly alkalizing. To derive the greatest benefits from dried fruits, look for produce that is free of sulfur, which is often used as a preservative in commercial brands. Since dried fruits also have a high natural sugar content, they should be eaten sparingly.

Cold-Pressed Oils. Cold-pressed oils are extracted without the use of excessive heat or chemicals. Some commercial methods of oil extraction not only destroy part of the oils' nutrient supply, but also cause the oils to break down during processing, making them harder for your body to digest and metabolize. Cold-pressed oils, however, retain all of their nutrients and are an important source of essential fatty acids (EFAs), which were first discussed in Chapter 2. (See page 21.)

EFAs are monounsaturated or polyunsaturated fats that are converted by the body into hormone-like substances known as prostaglandins, which regulate the body's inflammatory response, nourish the body fats used to strengthen cell walls and provide cellular energy, and enhance the immune system. Moreover, the EFAs found in cold-pressed oils help to bind and eliminate acids in the body.

Good sources of cold-pressed oils include borage, canola, evening primrose, flax, grape seed, and olive oil. Of these, only canola and olive oil should be used for cooking. The other oils can be added to foods after they have been prepared.

Herbs, Spices, and Salts. Herbs and spices have been used for centuries for their health-promoting properties. Most herbs and spices—including herbal teas—have an alkalizing effect on the body, as well.

Many herbs and spices, such as cayenne pepper, cinnamon, garlic, oregano, and sage, can add flavor to your meals. Unlike processed table salt (both iodized and noniodized), which should be avoided due to its acidifying effects, unprocessed sea salt and Celtic salt can also be used to spice up your meals. Both forms of these salts are alkalizing and are also rich in iodine, which is essential for healthy thyroid function.

Nuts. Earlier in this chapter (see page 83), you learned that most nuts are acidifying. The only alkalizing nuts are almonds and Brazil nuts. Brazil nuts are also a rich source of the trace mineral selenium, which is often lacking in the standard American diet and has been shown to have anti-cancer properties. Almond milk, made by combining purified water with almond paste, is an excellent alternative to dairy and soymilk because of its alkalizing effects.

Sprouts. Sprouts are a special class of food produced through the germination of beans, grains, and seeds. The germination process requires no soil—only water and warm room temperatures. In the sprouting process, even foods like beans and grains, which in their normal state are acidifying, become alkalizing as various changes occur. For example, during sprouting, proteins, fats, and starches are transformed into more easily digestible and assimilated amino acids, fatty acids, and vegetable sugars. In addition, sprouting increases the amounts of certain nutrients, especially the B vitamins. Sprouts are also energy-rich foods that are high in enzymes, proteins, vitamins, minerals, and other vital nutrients.

Although sprouts are now widely available in most health food stores and supermarkets across the country, I recommend that you learn how to make your own sprouted foods. (See the inset on page 89.) By growing your own sprouts, you can be assured of their freshness and have a constant supply of nutrient-rich, highly alkalizing foods readily available.

Vegetables. The foundation of every alkalizing meal is plenty of vegetables. These foods should always be included as part of your lunch and dinner, and when raw make an ideal snack food during the day. All vegetables are rich in vitamins, alkalizing minerals and salts, enzymes, phytonutrients (nutrients derived from plant foods), and fiber. But green vegetables—and especially leafy green vegetables—are also rich in chlorophyll, which is what gives them their green color. (Read the inset on page 90 to learn the relationship between chlorophyll and hemoglobin.)

Don't neglect vegetables of other colors, though. While not as rich in chlorophyll, they, too, are excellent sources of essential nutrients. Nongreen vegetables that you can eat freely include beets, green cabbage, carrots, cauliflower, garlic, onions, potatoes, radishes, red and yellow peppers, turnips, and squash.

Ideally, you should eat a certain amount of raw vegetables every day, while lightly steaming or sautéing the rest. This will ensure that the vegetables' rich supply of enzymes is not destroyed by overcooking. Enzymes are contained in all fresh fruits and vegetables and play an essential role in healthy digestion. When enzymes are deficient in your diet, your body is unable to properly digest and assimilate the foods you eat, setting the stage for further health problems.

How to Make Your Own Sprouts

It is very easy to sprout beans, grains, and seeds. All that is required are the foods themselves (preferably of organic grade), purified water, and a glass quart-size jar with a mesh top held in place by rubber bands.

To begin, select the type of food you wish to sprout and soak it for six to sixteen hours in purified water. (See the table below for specific soaking times.) The next morning, drain the beans, grains, or seeds and place them in the jar. Then place the jar in a warm, dry area. Twice a day, rinse the contents, pouring the water out through the mesh covering.

Depending on the bean, grain, or seed you choose, your sprouts will be ready for eating within forty-eight to seventy-two hours. Eat them soon thereafter, while they are still appealingly fresh and crisp. Whatever you don't eat, you can store in your refrigerator, where they will typically retain their freshness for up to a week. (If sprouts start to turn brown, as they so often are when they are purchased in a store, they are overripe and should not be eaten.) You can eat sprouts by themselves, you can liberally sprinkle them over salads, or you can add them to soups.

The following table will guide you in sprouting the food of your choice so that you can start making this nutritious, alkalizing food part of your daily diet.

SPROUTING DIRECTIONS			
TYPE OF SPROUT	SOAKING TIME	RINSES PER DAY	SPROUTING TIME
Alfalfa	6–8 hours	2 times per day	3 days
Chickpeas	16 hours	2–3 times per day	3 days
Lentils	8–12 hours	2 times per day	2–3 days
Mung beans	8–12 hours	2 times per day	2–3 days
Sesame seeds	8 hours	2 times per day	1–2 days
Sunflower seeds	6–8 hours	2 times per day	1–2 days

The Relationship Between Blood and Chlorophyll

One of the primary benefits of regularly consuming green vegetables is the supply of chlorophyll you receive as a result. Chlorophyll is often referred to as the "blood" of vegetables, and with good reason. The chemical makeup and molecular structure of this green pigment is closely related to that of hemoglobin, a prime component of human blood.

Hemoglobin is rich in iron, and plays an important role in delivering oxygen to your body's cells and tissues. In addition to iron, hemoglobin is composed of carbon, hydrogen, oxygen, and nitrogen. Chlorophyll is made up of the very same elements, except that it contains magnesium instead of iron.

The more chlorophyll-rich vegetables you consume each day, the more you will enhance your body's ability to transport oxygen to all of your cells and tissues, for this is exactly what chlorophyll does once the green vegetables you eat are digested and metabolized. Chlorophyll also helps the liver and other organs detoxify, and prevents carcinogens from binding to cellular DNA. It aids in the breakdown and elimination of calcium stones, as well. This is of particular importance to people who are overly acidic, since calcium stones often form as a result of the body's attempts to neutralize excess acid buildup. Considering all of these health-producing benefits, you can clearly see why green vegetables should be an important part of your daily diet.

Be aware that enzymes are inactivated and destroyed when vegetables are cooked in temperatures over 118°F. (You will learn more about enzymes in Chapter 6.)

Whenever possible, it is a good idea to select organically grown vegetables, which contain more abundant amounts of essential nutrients than commercially grown produce, and are also free of pesticides and a variety of other harmful chemicals. Organic vegetables are now readily available in health food stores and many commercial supermarket chains, as well. You can also find them at your local farm stands and farmers' markets. Whether you use organic or nonorganic produce, always be sure to wash the vegetables thoroughly before eating them.

If you suffer from sugar sensitivities and/or are hyper- or hypo-glycemic, initially you may want to avoid vegetables that have a naturally high sugar content, such as beets and carrots. Over time, however, as your health improves and your sugar problems stabilize, these vegetables can be added back to your diet and eaten in moderation.

Alkalizing foods should compose the largest part of every meal and snack you consume throughout the day. Especially concentrate on generous amounts of green, leafy vegetables, and consider adding sprouts to your menu to speed your return to a healthy acid-alkaline balance. Also be sure to drink adequate amounts of purified water or mineral water with a pH greater than 7.0. The charts in the next section will make it easier for you to choose your foods wisely.

The Humble Potato—
An Often Overlooked Alkalizing Vegetable

Historically, potatoes have been a staple food in every culture in which they have been available. But with all the emphasis today on "low-carb" diets, many people are eliminating potatoes from their diets, along with cereals and grains. This is a big mistake if you need to shift your pH levels to a more alkaline state.

Unlike cereals and grains, which for the most part have an acidifying effect on the body, potatoes are very high in alkalizing nutrients. So alkalizing are potatoes that many native healers and naturopathic physicians recommend potato juice as a first resort for relieving ulcers and stomach problems caused by over-acidity. Potato skins are also a rich source of vitamin C, and potatoes can help fuel your body's energy supply, as well.

Unfortunately, in today's standard American diet, the health-giving properties of potatoes are often destroyed through unhealthy means of preparation. Even when they are not transformed into French fries, an extremely acidic junk food, potatoes are often buried beneath heaps of sour cream, another acidifying substance. By contrast, baked or boiled potatoes or yams served with a small dollop of organic butter or cold-pressed olive oil—along with a dash of herbs or spices, perhaps—makes a nutritious side dish. Just as important, properly prepared potatoes have potent alkalizing benefits.

ALKALIZING AND ACIDIFYING FOOD CHARTS

The following tables categorize the foods groups discussed in this chapter according to the degree—strong or mild—of alkalinity or acidity they produce in the body. Your goal is to create a daily diet that will optimize your body's ability to create and maintain proper acid-alkaline balance. To do this, you will want to eat as many of the alkalizing foods as you desire throughout the day, while minimizing your intake of acidifying foods, initially making them no more than 20 percent of your total food intake. Obviously, it makes good sense to eat a lot of foods classified as strongly alkalizing, especially if you are suffering from chronic acidosis. These foods will produce more powerful alkalizing effects than foods that are only mildly alkalizing. Conversely, you will want to eat sparingly of foods that are strongly acidifying, choosing your acidifying foods from those that are only mildly so.

THE pH EFFECT OF VEGETABLES				
VEGETABLE	STRONGLY ACIDIFYING	MILDLY ACIDIFYING	MILDLY ALKALIZING	STRONGLY ALKALIZING
Artichokes				X
Asparagus			X	
Beets and Beet Greens				X
Broccoli				X
Brussels Sprouts				X
Carrots				X
Cauliflower			X	
Chicory				X
Cucumber				X
Dandelion Greens				X
Endives			X	
Escarole				X
Garlic			X	
Green Beans				X
Green Cabbage				X

	Strongly Acidifying	Mildly Acidifying	Mildly Alkalizing	Strongly Alkalizing
Lettuce (avoid iceberg)				■
Onions			■	
Potatoes				■
Radishes			■	
Red Cabbage				■
Shallots			■	
Spinach				■
Squash				■
Sweet Peppers				■
Sweet Potatoes				■
Turnips			■	
Yams				■
Zucchini				■

THE pH EFFECT OF GRAINS

GRAIN	STRONGLY ACIDIFYING	MILDLY ACIDIFYING	MILDLY ALKALIZING	STRONGLY ALKALIZING
Amaranth		■		
Barley		■		
Buckwheat		■		
Bulgur		■		
Millet	■			
Oats		■		
Quinoa		■		
Rice, Brown		■		
Rice, White	■			
Rye		■		
Spelt		■		
Wheat, Semolina	■			
Wheat, White	■			
Wheat, Whole		■		

THE pH EFFECT OF BREADS

Bread	Strongly Acidifying	Mildly Acidifying	Mildly Alkalizing	Strongly Alkalizing
Dark Bread (Pumpernickel, etc.) (Yeast Free)		X		
White Bread	X			
Whole-Grain Bread (Yeast Free)		X		
Yeast Bread	X			

THE pH EFFECT OF DAIRY PRODUCTS

Dairy Product	Strongly Acidifying	Mildly Acidifying	Mildly Alkalizing	Strongly Alkalizing
Butter, heated	X			
Butter, raw, fresh			X	
Buttermilk, fresh			X	
Cheese, Provolone		X		
Cheese, sharp (Cheddar, Parmesan, etc.)	X			
Cheese, soft (Brie, Camembert, etc.)		X		
Cheese, Swiss		X		
Egg Yolk			X	
Eggs, whole		X		
Kefir	X			
Milk, pasteurized		X		
Milk, raw whole			X	
Whey, fresh			X	
Yogurt, plain, organic		X		
Yogurt, sweetened	X			

THE pH EFFECT OF MEATS, POULTRY, AND FISH

Meat, Poultry, Fish	Strongly Acidifying	Mildly Acidifying	Mildly Alkalizing	Strongly Alkalizing
Beef	■			
Carp	■			
Chicken		■		
Cold Cuts/Processed Meats	■			
Crayfish	■			
Flounder		■		
Herring	■			
Lamb	■			
Lobster	■			
Mackerel	■			
Oysters		■		
Perch		■		
Pork	■			
Salmon	■			
Sole		■		
Trout		■		

THE pH EFFECT OF LEGUMES

Legume	Strongly Acidifying	Mildly Acidifying	Mildly Alkalizing	Strongly Alkalizing
Chickpeas (Garbanzo Beans)	■			
Kidney Beans		■		
Lentils		■		
Navy Beans		■		
Peanuts	■			
Peas		■		
Soybeans	■			
White Beans		■		

THE pH EFFECT OF NUTS AND SEEDS

Nut or Seed	Strongly Acidifying	Mildly Acidifying	Mildly Alkalizing	Strongly Alkalizing
Almonds				■
Brazil Nuts			■	
Cashews		■		
Coconuts				
Hazelnuts	■			
Pecans	■			
Pine Nuts		■		
Pistachio Nuts	■			
Pumpkin Seeds	■			
Sesame Seeds		■		
Sunflower Seeds	■			
Walnuts	■			

THE pH EFFECT OF FRUIT

Fruit	Strongly Acidifying	Mildly Acidifying	Mildly Alkalizing	Strongly Alkalizing
Apples		■		
Apricots, fresh		■		
Avocados			■	
Bananas			■	
Black Currants	■			
Blackthorn Berries	■			
Blueberries		■		
Cherries, Bing		■		
Figs, fresh		■		
Grapefruit			■	
Grapes		■		
Kiwis	■			
Lemons				■
Limes				■

	Strongly Acidifying	Mildly Acidifying	Mildly Alkalizing	Strongly Alkalizing
Mandarin Oranges	▓			
Mangos		▓		
Melons		▓		
Mulberries	▓			
Nectarines	▓			
Oranges	▓			
Pears, Bartlett and Bosc		▓		
Persimmons		▓		
Pineapples	▓			
Plums		▓		
Pomegranates		▓		
Raspberries	▓			
Red Currants	▓			
Strawberries, sweet		▓		
Strawberries, tart	▓			
Tomatoes, uncooked			▓	
Watermelon		▓		

THE pH EFFECT OF DRIED FRUIT				
Dried Fruit	Strongly Acidifying	Mildly Acidifying	Mildly Alkalizing	Strongly Alkalizing
Apples		▓		
Apricots			▓	
Bananas			▓	
Dates			▓	
Figs		▓		
Mangos		▓		
Peaches		▓		
Pears		▓		
Pineapples		▓		
Prunes		▓		
Raisins			▓	

THE pH EFFECT OF BEVERAGES

Beverage	Strongly Acidifying	Mildly Acidifying	Mildly Alkalizing	Strongly Alkalizing
Almond Milk			■	
Beer		■		
Black Tea	■			
Cocoa	■			
Coffee	■			
Herbal Teas			■	
Hot Chocolate	■			
Liquor	■			
Milk	■			
Soda	■			
Vegetable Juice (freshly made)				■
Water, Mineral (carbonated)		■		
Water, Mineral (heavily carbonated)	■			
Water, Mineral (noncarbonated)			■	
Water, Spring or Filtered			■	
Water, Tap	■			
Whiskey	■			
Wine	■			

THE pH EFFECT OF FATS AND OILS

Fat or Oil	Strongly Acidifying	Mildly Acidifying	Mildly Alkalizing	Strongly Alkalizing
Butter			■	
Cold-Pressed, Unrefined Oils (heated), such as canola, olive, etc.		■		

	Strongly Acidifying	Mildly Acidifying	Mildly Alkalizing	Strongly Alkalizing
Cold-Pressed, Unrefined Oils (unheated), such as canola, olive, etc.			■	
Hydrogenated Fats	■			
Lard	■			
Margarine	■			
Nonhydrogenated Fats			■	
Peanut Oil	■			
Walnut Oil	■			

THE pH EFFECT OF CONDIMENTS, HERBS, AND SPICES

Condiment, Herb, Spice	Strongly Acidifying	Mildly Acidifying	Mildly Alkalizing	Strongly Alkalizing
Apple Cider Vinegar				■
Herbs			■	
Ketchup	■			
Mayonnaise	■			
Mustard, Commercial	■			
Mustard, Organic		■		
Pickles	■			
Salt, Celtic and Sea			■	
Salt, Processed	■			
Spices			■	
Sugar	■			
Vinegars Other Than Apple Cider	■			

FOOD COMBINING TIPS

To enhance the health benefits provided by my pH Factor diet, I would like to add a few comments about food combining. The principles of food combining are based on the fact that each food you eat is digested according to the nature of that specific food group. For example, when you eat foods that are primarily high in protein, such as meat, fish, or poultry, they are digested primarily in the stomach.

To do so effectively, your body needs to temporarily create a highly acidic environment. By contrast, when you eat foods that are high in starchy carbohydrates, such as breads, potatoes, or yams, your body begins to digest them in the mouth as they are chewed, and completes the process in the small intestines. For this function to occur, a mildly alkaline environment is required.

Based on the above, it makes sense to avoid combining protein-rich foods with starchy carbohydrate foods during mealtime. By eating such foods together, the body is forced to attempt two entirely opposite tasks—digesting the protein foods in a highly acidic environment, while simultaneously digesting the starchy carbohydrates in an environment that is mildly alkaline. This simply isn't possible. As a result, when eaten together, both food groups usually end up partially undigested. This means that your body is not able obtain the full supply of nutrients offered by the foods. Moreover, the undigested remnants start to build up in the colon, where they decompose and ferment, creating toxins and mucus.

Below, you will find basic guidelines for food combining. Follow these rules, and you'll find it easy to design meals that are truly healthful.

❏ Do not combine protein-rich foods (meats, fish, poultry, and dairy) with starchy carbohydrates (potatoes, yams, breads, wheat products, and grain products). Note that this guideline eliminates not only a meal of steak and potatoes, but also several common lunch staples such as chicken salad, roast beef, tuna fish, and turkey sandwiches.

❏ Feel free to combine nonstarchy carbohydrate vegetables (green leafy vegetables, as well as other vegetables) with either protein-rich foods or starchy carbohydrates. Such vegetables will not interfere with the digestion of either food group.

❏ As far as possible, eat fruits alone rather than with meals. The only exceptions to this rule are avocados and tomatoes, both of which can be included with meals.

❏ Avoid drinking water with your meals—especially when the meal features protein-rich foods—so as not to dilute the digestive juices needed to break down solid foods. Water is best consumed twenty minutes before eating, or sixty minutes afterwards.

❏ To further aid your body's digestive process, be sure to chew your food thoroughly before swallowing.

CONCLUSION

As this chapter has shown, the over-acidity that plagues our nation today has its roots in the many acidifying foods that make up the standard American diet. By simply changing your diet to one that emphasizes alkalizing foods and following the guidelines presented in this chapter, you can significantly reduce the toxic burden of acidosis both easily and safely. It may take time before you see the results you are looking for—greater energy and freedom from disease symptoms—but with a little patience and discipline, you can join my many clients who have turned their health around by making simple dietary changes.

While the foods you eat are of paramount importance, certain nutritional supplements can further help you regain and maintain optimal acid-alkaline balance. You'll learn more about these supplements in Chapter 6.

6

Supplementation— The Extra Edge

The dietary guidelines outlined in the previous chapter should serve as your primary means of restoring and maintaining optimal acid-alkaline balance. But for most people, I also recommend the use of nutritional supplements. In this chapter, I will share with you the most important nutrients you can use to enhance your overall health and aid in your recovery from over-acidity. First, though, let's discuss why nutritional supplementation is so important.

Even if you eat fresh, organically grown food at all of your meals—a difficult feat for many people—such foods, although certainly richer in nutrients than standard commercial foods, are probably still incapable of meeting all of your nutritional needs. One reason for this is the nature of modern life. Every day, we are bombarded by stressors in the forms of difficult relationships, both at home and at work; noise and air pollution; and invading pathogens such as bacteria, fungi, and viruses. Some of us do a good job of managing the stress caused by such factors, but the one stressor to which we are all susceptible is chemical stress.

According to Drs. Robert Ivker and Robert Anderson, "Chemical stress may come from polluted air and water, food pesticides, insecticides, heavy metals, and even radioactive wastes. More than ever before, foreign chemicals can be found in our foods and environment. Many of these are commercially synthesized, but quite a few are naturally occurring as well." Your continued exposure to chemical stressors places a constant burden on your body as it works to maintain homeostasis. Because of this burden, the nutrients available from the foods you eat, as well as those that your body has stored, can quickly become depleted. For this reason alone, daily supplementation with nutrients is a good idea.

But the challenge of meeting your body's nutritional needs does not end there. Adding to the problem of stressors is the fact that the soil in which food crops are now grown contains significantly reduced levels of vital trace minerals. Because of the commercial farming methods used by today's agricultural industry, much of the trace minerals that had been abundant in our topsoil prior to the mid-twentieth century have been greatly depleted. This has resulted in significant declines in the overall nutrient content of the foods grown on our farms.

Compounding the problem is the fact that much of our modern-day food supply takes weeks or even months to reach us once it has been harvested. Very few of us eat locally grown food these days. Instead, the food that we consume, even if grown organically, is often shipped from other parts of the country, frozen, and warehoused along the way. This further reduces the nutrient content of food.

The final reason that I recommend supplementation, of course, has to do with the burden of over-acidity that so many of us currently face. As we have discussed previously, to cope with over-acidity, your body draws from its stored mineral supplies, using those minerals to buffer and neutralize the effects of toxic acid buildup. The result is not only over-acidity, but also nutritional deficiencies.

With all of these factors working against us, you can understand why I feel that nutritional supplementation is so important. Now let's take a look at the nutrients and other supplements I strongly recommend as part of your daily health regimen.

ESSENTIAL NUTRIENTS FOR MAINTAINING PROPER pH BALANCE

To aid you in your journey to optimal health, I recommend daily supplementation of the following select group of vitamins, minerals, essential fatty acids, and digestive enzymes, along with the sulfur-compound MSM and green drinks. When purchasing these supplements, choose brands composed of food-grade concentrates—supplements containing nutrients derived from natural foods and herbs—as the body can use them more easily than it can synthetic brands. A number of manufacturers provide food-grade multivitamin/multimineral formulas that offer adequate amounts of the vitamins and minerals listed below. Read labels for more information, noting the amount of each nutrient included, and checking to see if unnecessary fillers, dyes, and other nonessential ingredients have been used. Once you are satisfied with the supplement's quality, follow the manufacturer's directions for best results. (To learn more about reading a supplement label, see the inset below.)

How to Read a Supplement Label

Before purchasing a nutritional supplement, it is important to understand the quality of the product you are considering. One of the best ways to get the information you need is to read the product label. Here are some guidelines for doing so.

Dietary supplements include vitamins, minerals, herbs, "green drinks," essential fatty acids (EFAs), and other nutrients derived or synthesized from food sources. According to the Dietary Supplement Health and Education Act (DSHEA) of 1994, such supplements are not considered drugs and therefore are not required to be reviewed by the Food and Drug Administration (FDA) before entering the marketplace. However, the FDA can and often does regulate the claims that supplement manufacturers can make about their products.

Typically, product labels consist of a statement of identity, a structure-function claim, the form of product and net contents, directions for use, a supplement facts panel, a listing of "other ingredients," and the name and address of the manufacturer. Let's look at each of these in turn.

In the *statement of identity,* you should find the brand name of the product and wording that clearly identifies the product as a "dietary supplement." This is followed by the *structure-function claim,* which explains the health benefits of the nutrients included in the product, along with a required disclaimer saying, "This statement has not been evaluated by the Food and Drug Administration. This product is not intended to diagnose, treat, cure, or prevent any disease." Structure-function claims cannot say that a product or nutrient treats a disease, so be wary of any products for which such claims are made. But structure-function claims can state the role or function of the nutrient or nutrients in the body. For example, a multivitamin/multimineral formula with a structure function claim stating "Helps support immune function" is perfectly acceptable. The federally required disclaimer means exactly what it says—that the FDA has not evaluated the claim, and that no diagnostic, treatment, prevention, or curative claims can be made about the product in question. This is simply a formality in accordance with the DSHEA legislation.

Quite simply, the *form of product and net contents* tells you the form the product is in and the amount of its contents. Products can come in a variety of forms, such as capsules, tablets, liquids, or powders. If capsule or tablet forms are used, the label should tell you the number of capsules or tablets included. If the product is in liquid or powder form, the total weight (usually ounces) will be listed.

The *directions for use* tell you how the product is intended to be taken. For example, the label may say, "Take one capsule daily." Be sure that you don't exceed the recommended serving size.

You'll want to pay particular attention to the *supplement facts panel*. There, you will find the listed serving size—e.g., one tablet, one capsule, etc.—as well as the product's active ingredients, along with the amount of each ingredient per serving and the total percentage of the Daily Value—recommended daily intake—the product supplies for each nutrient. If an asterisk follows any of the ingredients, this means that no Daily Value has been established for that particular nutrient.

The *other ingredients* list tells you which nonnutritive (inactive) ingredients were used in the formulation and manufacture of the product. Such ingredients are presented in descending order, based on how much of each ingredient was used, with the ingredient present in the largest amount listed first, and the ingredient present in the smallest amount listed last. Common substances found in this listing include gelatin, water, binders, fillers, and coatings. Ideally, the product you choose should not contain the last three types of substances.

Finally, the label should supply you with the name and address of the product's manufacturer or distributor, including the zip code and, ideally, a telephone number or website through which you can contact the company. If the product you are considering does not include all of the above information, I advise you to avoid purchasing it. And definitely be suspicious of any product that comes with a label claiming it can cure or treat a specific disease condition.

Essential Vitamins

Vitamins are groups of substances essential for normal metabolism, growth and development, and the regulation of cell function. For the most part, vitamins cannot be manufactured by the body, and therefore must be obtained daily through diet and supplementation. The most important vitamins with regard to proper acid-alkaline balance are vitamins A, B_6, B_{12}, C, and D, and folic acid.

Vitamin A

Vitamin A is required for the proper metabolism of calcium, a mineral with highly alkalizing properties. Vitamin A is also necessary to ensure good health of the eyes, skin, and teeth, and plays a key role in bone growth, cell differentiation, and tissue repair. It is also a potent antioxidant and important for proper immune function and protection against infectious disease.

Both stress and disease can diminish vitamin A stores, as can alcohol consumption, which we know also has a significant acidifying effect on the body. Signs of vitamin A deficiency include night blindness, impaired bone and teeth formation, impaired immunity, and inflammation of the eyes.

It is best to take vitamin A in the form of beta-carotene, which your body can convert to vitamin A in the liver. Beta-carotene is abundant in many vegetables, all of which are alkalizing, but since studies have found that nearly a third of the American public consumes less than 65 percent of the Daily Value for vitamin A, I suggest supplementing with between 5,000 to 8,000 international units of beta-carotene each day.

Vitamin B_6

Vitamin B_6, also known as pyridoxine, is involved in a wide range of processes, including immune function, energy production, hemoglobin production, and the synthesis of proteins from amino acids. With regard to acid-alkaline balance, vitamin B_6 plays two important roles. First, it helps regulate your body's sodium-potassium balance, which, as we saw in Chapter 4, is essential for optimal energy production at the cellular level. An imbalance in sodium-potassium levels can have wide-ranging negative health effects and can contribute to acidosis. Second, vitamin B_6 is required for the production of

hydrochloric acid (HCL), which helps your body digest and metabolize protein foods, and also aids in the absorption of calcium. (For
more information about HCL, see page 45.)

Because it is water-soluble—which means that it cannot be stored
by the body—supplies of vitamin B_6 can quickly be diminished.
Signs of B_6 deficiency include anemia, fatigue, headache, insomnia,
muscle cramps and spasms, and nerve malfunctions.

Although this vitamin is found in a variety of foods, such as
bananas, cabbage, cauliflower, eggs, fish, poultry, organ meats, and
whole grains, it is often destroyed by commercial food processing
and storage. That's why I recommend taking 2 milligrams each day,
ideally as part of an overall vitamin B formula.

Vitamin B$_{12}$

Healthy bones are a sign that your body's pH levels are in balance,
whereas bone loss is a sure indication of over-acidity. Vitamin B_{12} is
essential if the cells that build bones are to carry out their functions.
Signs of vitamin B_{12} deficiency include pernicious anemia, dizziness,
fatigue, gastrointestinal disorders, low blood pressure, memory
problems, moodiness, numbness, and vision problems.

The best food sources of vitamin B_{12} are meats, fish, and dairy products. Vegetarians are often deficient in vitamin B_{12} since it is not found
in significant amounts in fruits and vegetables. Since you, too, will be
limiting your consumption of such foods in order to achieve proper pH
balance, it is a good idea to take daily supplements of vitamin B_{12}. I recommend that you take at least 3 micrograms of B_{12} per day.

Vitamin C

Vitamin C, also known as ascorbic acid, is one of the most important
nutrients that your body requires because of the many varied
processes in which it plays a key role. Besides being a potent antioxidant, it is essential for proper immune function and contributes to
the health of bones, blood vessels, cartilage, joint linings, ligaments,
skin, teeth, and vertebrae. It also is needed for proper wound healing, plays an important part in your body's detoxification processes,
and enhances calcium absorption.

For all of its important functions, vitamin C is one of the least stable vitamins, and can neither be manufactured nor stored by the body.
Therefore, it is crucial that you consume an adequate amount of vita-

min C each and every day. Signs of vitamin C deficiency are numerous, and include anemia, bleeding gums, increased tendency to bruise, lowered resistance to infections, mouth ulcers, and slow wound healing.

The best food sources of vitamin C include cherries, citrus fruits, dark green and leafy vegetables, green and red peppers, papaya, parsley, potato skins, and strawberries. It is not found in any dairy, fish, poultry, or meat products.

Currently, the recommended daily intake of vitamin C is 60 milligrams, but most holistic health practitioners regard that amount as being extremely low. I advise you to take 3,000 milligrams of vitamin C per day, divided into three doses of 1,000 milligrams each spread throughout the day.

Vitamin D

Vitamin has recently been determined to act more like a hormone than a vitamin. It occurs in ten forms (D_1 to D_{10}), but the two most important forms are D_2 and D_3.

Vitamin D helps to maintain a healthy acid-alkaline balance by aiding in the absorption of calcium and regulating the metabolism of both calcium and phosphorus. In doing so, it also enhances the health of your bones and teeth. Vitamin D also helps regulate the nervous system, maintain the health of the cardiovascular system, and maintain normal blood clot function.

Good food sources of vitamin D include butter, cod liver oil, egg yolk, liver, milk, and oily fish such as herring, mackerel, sardines, and salmon. In addition, regular exposure to sunlight can help your body manufacture its own vitamin D supply. Because most people's lifestyle affords them little time outdoors, though, they are often unknowingly deficient in vitamin D. Signs of vitamin D deficiency include bone softening (osteomalacia), hearing loss, nearsightedness, osteoporosis, psoriasis, and tetany (a form of muscle spasm).

To help ensure that you get the vitamin D you need, try to expose at least a third of your body—your arms, face, and hands—to sunlight for twenty to thirty minutes each day. As a supplement, take between 200 to 400 international units per day.

Folic Acid

Folic acid—also known as folate, folacin, and vitamin B_9—aids in the production of red blood cells, helps to regulate proper cell division, is needed to properly metabolize sugars, and is needed for the production of neurotransmitters. It also plays a key role in helping to rid the bones of homocysteine, an amino acid that has been associated with both artherosclerosis and osteoporosis.

The best food sources for folic acid are dark green vegetables, eggs, nuts, and organ meats. Signs of deficiency include anemia, diarrhea, fatigue, gastrointestinal disorders, headache, irritability, palpitations, and general weakness. Research shows that folic acid deficiency is quite common, due to such factors as poor diet, drug and alcohol abuse, and stress. I therefore recommend supplementing with 400 micrograms each day, preferably as part of an overall vitamin B formula.

Essential Minerals

As discussed earlier in the chapter, over the years, commercial farming methods have greatly depleted the minerals found in our soil and, as a consequence, in our fruits, vegetables, and grains. This trend began in the early 1900s, and in 1936 was of sufficient significance to be noted in U.S. Senate Document No. 264:

> The alarming fact is that foods (fruits, vegetables and grains) now being raised on millions of acres of land that no longer contains enough of certain minerals are starving us—no matter how much we eat. No man of today can eat enough fruits and vegetables to supply his system with the minerals he requires for perfect health because his stomach isn't big enough to hold them. The truth is that our foods vary enormously in value, and some of them aren't worth eating as food. . . . Our physical well-being is more directly dependent upon the minerals we take into our system than upon calories or vitamins or upon the precise proportions of starch, protein, or carbohydrates we consume.

Minerals play many vital roles in the body, working in conjunction with vitamins, enzymes, hormones, and other nutrient cofactors to regulate numerous biological functions, from proper blood formation to energy production to nerve transmission. Minerals are also key in the regulation of a healthy acid-alkaline balance. The most important minerals in this regard are boron, calcium, copper, magnesium, phosphorus, potassium, silica, and zinc.

Boron

Boron is important to acid-alkaline balance because it helps the body metabolize and make use of various other nutrients, such as calcium, vitamin D, and magnesium, all of which play roles in maintaining healthy pH levels. Boron also contributes to the overall health of the bones, which is where your body stores much of the minerals it uses to buffer and neutralize acid buildup. Recent research also suggests that boron helps regulate your body's endocrine system, which is responsible for producing hormones.

Potential signs of boron deficiency include diminished levels of the hormones estrogen and testosterone, both of which are essential for healthy bones, and osteoporosis. Among older women, boron deficiency can also contribute to problems related to postmenopause.

Currently, there is no established daily requirement for boron intake. Fortunately, adequate levels of boron can be obtained solely from your diet through plentiful amounts of fruits, nuts, and vegetables. I recommend this approach over supplementation because taking more than 3 milligrams of boron in supplement form can interfere with the body's ability to make use of its calcium supplies. However, no problem is caused when even higher levels of boron are obtained directly from foods.

Calcium

Calcium is the most abundant mineral in the body. Nearly all of it—99 percent—is stored in bone tissue, where it is used to ensure the health of both bones and teeth. Your body uses the remaining 1 percent of its calcium supply to help regulate blood clotting and blood pressure levels, cardiovascular function, cell division, and muscle and nerve function. Calcium is also required for healthy skin. Finally, it is one of the primary acid-buffering minerals called upon by your body whenever excess acids pose a problem.

It is important to supply your body with adequate amounts of calcium each and every day, ideally through a combination of diet and supplementation. Unfortunately, the standard American diet has been shown to be severely lacking in calcium. This is not surprising given the chronic state of acidosis such a diet creates.

The most familiar signs of calcium deficiency are bone and skeletal problems. Of these, the most common are fracture and osteoporosis. Other symptoms include anxiety, brittle nails, depression, insomnia, muscle cramps, diminished nerve function, and problems related to the teeth.

According to Dr. Susan Brown, a leading medical anthropologist, Americans derive 80 percent of their calcium from dairy foods. In other parts of the world, however, the primary sources of dietary calcium are vegetables—especially broccoli, collard greens, and dark green leafy vegetables—and certain types of fish, such as sardines and salmon. Almonds and Brazil nuts, both of which are also alkalizing foods, are other good food sources of calcium. Dr. Brown reports that calcium derived from nondairy sources is far more absorbable than calcium derived from dairy products, and therefore meets a greater percentage of your body's daily calcium needs. Given that fact, as well as the acidifying effect of a diet high in dairy products, I strongly suggest that you make vegetables your primary food source of calcium, along with nuts and fish.

Unfortunately, even a diet rich in calcium will not necessarily meet all of your daily calcium needs. In fact, research shows that calcium deficiency is widespread in this country. Therefore, supplementing with calcium, in addition to regularly eating calcium-rich foods, makes good sense. For best results, use a food-grade multivitamin/multimineral formula that contains twice as much calcium as magnesium—1,000 to 1,500 milligrams of calcium to 500 to 750 milligrams of magnesium. This ratio will optimize your body's ability to absorb both nutrients.

Copper

Copper is an essential trace mineral that is found in all body tissues, and is especially concentrated in the liver and brain. Among its various functions, copper helps the body absorb and use iron to synthesize hemoglobin. It also plays a role in the regulation of insulin levels and helps prevent unhealthy weight gain. Recently, scientists discovered that copper is necessary for healthy bones, as well.

Despite its importance to good health, copper is one of the most noticeably lacking minerals in the standard American diet, which contains only about 50 percent of the recommended daily intake of copper. Symptoms of copper deficiency include anemia, dermatitis, edema, chronic fatigue, impaired respiration, and tissue and blood vessel damage.

Like boron, copper is best obtained through food sources, since the recommended daily amount is only 1.5 to 3 milligrams. The best food sources of copper include dark leafy green vegetables, eggs, lamb, legumes, pecans, oysters, poultry, and walnuts. In order to help create proper pH balance, I recommend making dark leafy green vegetables a staple food source.

Magnesium

Approximately 65 percent of the body's magnesium stores are found in bones and teeth, followed by high concentrations in muscles. Magnesium is also contained in blood and other body fluids.

Magnesium plays many roles in the body, including participating in hundreds of enzymatic reactions and acting as a musculoskeletal relaxant. Magnesium is also important for the health of the heart, as it appears to affect the muscle tone of the blood vessels. It also aids in proper cell division, cell maintenance and repair, energy production, hormone regulation, nerve transmission, protein metabolism, and thyroid function. Moreover, this mineral helps the body assimilate and use calcium and vitamin D, and is necessary for healthy bones and teeth.

Although often undiagnosed, magnesium deficiency is very common among Americans due to a variety of factors, such as poor diet, mineral-deficient crops, the overcooking of foods, and the overconsumption of alcohol. Symptoms of magnesium deficiency include depression, fatigue, gastrointestinal disorders, hypertension, irregular heartbeat, memory problems, mood swings, impaired motor skills, muscle spasms, nausea, and osteoporosis.

The best dietary sources of magnesium are dark green vegetables, which are also highly alkalizing and rich in chlorophyll. Other good food sources include apricots, avocados, brown rice, legumes, nuts, and seeds. As a dietary supplement, magnesium is best taken as part of a food-grade multivitamin/mineral supplement that also contains calcium. I recommend a daily intake of 500 to 750 milligrams of magnesium in conjunction with 1,000 to 1,500 milligrams of calcium.

Phosphorus

Phosphorus is the second most abundant mineral in the body, exceeded only by calcium. Like calcium, it is primarily concentrated in the bones and teeth, although it is found in every body cell. It is involved in nearly all of the body's biochemical reactions. Among its many functions, phosphorus helps form DNA and RNA; aids in cell communication, growth, and repair; and plays a vital role in energy production. It also is essential for good bone and teeth health, heart function, muscle and nerve function, and the metabolism of B vitamins, calcium, fat, glucose, and starch. Finally, it is one of the most important minerals that your body draws upon to buffer and neutralize acid buildup, and therefore is essential for proper pH balance.

Although phosphorus deficiency is considered rare, phosphorus stores can easily be depleted due to the use of antacids and a lack of vitamin D—a vitamin needed for the absorption and storage of phosphorus. Symptoms of phosphorus deficiency include anxiety, arthritis, impaired bone growth, irritability, and general weakness. Health problems can also occur when phosphorous levels exceed those of calcium and, conversely, when levels of phosphorous are low compared with those of calcium. For optimal health, phosphorus and calcium levels should be in a 1–to–1 ratio. However, most people, especially those who follow the standard American diet, have far more phosphorus than calcium.

The best food sources of phosphorus are protein-rich foods such as cheese, eggs, fish, milk, meats, and poultry. Nuts, seeds, and whole grains are other good sources. Given the rarity of phosphorus deficiencies, I recommend that you obtain phosphorus from your diet, but I caution against consuming too much protein-rich food due to its acidifying effects. By following the 80–to–20 percent alkaline-to-acid rule discussed in Chapter 5, you can avoid this problem.

Potassium

Potassium is an essential body salt. Approximately 98 percent of your body's potassium stores are found within the cell walls, where this mineral regulates water and acid-alkaline balance, making it crucial for proper pH levels. Potassium also helps conduct bioelectrical current throughout the body, maintains cellular integrity and fluid balance, helps regulate nerve function, and aids in energy production and heart function.

Potassium deficiency is quite common among most Americans—especially among our aging population and among people who suffer from chronic illness. One of the main causes of potassium deficiency, besides poor diet, is our nation's overreliance on diuretics and laxatives, both of which strip potassium from the body. Eating canned and processed foods can also deplete potassium supplies through an excessive consumption of salt. Symptoms of potassium deficiency include arrhythmia, depression, fatigue, hypertension, hyperglycemia, mood swings, and impaired nerve function.

The best food sources of potassium are fresh fruits and vegetables. Bananas, in particular, are rich in potassium. Other good sources include nuts, seeds, whole grains, and fish such as salmon and sardines. Though there is no established recommended daily allowance for potassium, most people require between 2,000 and 5,000 milligrams per day. A variety of potassium supplements are available in both tablet and liquid form. Both of these forms are well absorbed.

Silica

Silica, also known as silicon, is the most abundant mineral on earth. In your body, it is primarily concentrated in the arteries, collagen, connective tissue, eyes, hair, ligaments, nails, skin, teeth, and tendons. Silica is important to pH balance because it helps make other minerals, particularly calcium, more bioavailable, ensuring that adequate calcium stores are present when the body needs to draw upon them to buffer and neutralize acid buildup.

Signs of silica deficiency include atherosclerosis, fatigue, lowered resistance to infectious disease, diminished strength of bones and teeth, lessened elasticity of skin, and joint problems.

Silica is widely available in the fibers of most fresh fruits and vegetables, grains, nuts, and seeds. However, since fibers are stripped during commercial food processing, people who eat a diet high in processed foods are usually deficient in silica. A recommended daily allowance for silica has not been established, but research indicates that at least 20 to 30 milligrams of silica per day is required to maintain good health.

Zinc

Zinc is one of the most important minerals needed for good health. In addition to being a potent antioxidant, zinc is necessary for the performance of over two hundred enzymatic reactions. It also is important for detoxification, bone repair, maintaining healthy cellular membranes and tissues, ensuring proper immune function, and regulating insulin production. Zinc also helps your body absorb and utilize vitamins A and D and calcium. In men, zinc is essential for the health of the prostate gland.

Zinc deficiencies are quite common in the United States—especially among vegetarians. Lack of zinc can result in dermatitis, fatigue, hair loss, impaired immune function, loss of libido, and osteoporosis. It can also increase the risk of prostate problems, including enlargement, infection, and cancer of the prostate. The recommended daily allowance for zinc is 15 milligrams for adults, although many health researchers believe this level is far too low. I recommend 30 to 45 milligrams per day, especially for men over forty years of age.

The best dietary sources of zinc include beef, egg yolks, herring, nuts, and shellfish. Whole grain bread also contains zinc. However, given the large number of people who suffer from wheat allergies or sensitivities, bread is not an optimum food source—especially because breads are also highly acidifying. When supplementing with zinc, it is best to take it in the form of picolinate for optimum absorption. Since zinc can interfere with your body's ability to absorb and utilize copper, you'll want to take these supplements at different times of the day.

Essential Fatty Acids

Although excess fat consumption can lead to a variety of health problems, your body requires certain types of fat each day in order to function properly. Those healthful fats that are not produced by your body, and therefore must be obtained through diet and supplementation, are known as *essential fatty acids* (EFAs).

EFAs help your body produce energy, regulate hormone and nerve function, and maintain healthy brain function. They also aid in overall musculoskeletal function and calcium metabolism, and help to reduce inflammation in the body. EFAs make up part of cell membranes and are particularly concentrated in the adrenal glands, brain cells, eyes, nerve cells, and sex glands. But perhaps EFAs are best known for helping to maintain cardiac health by reducing cholesterol, low-density lipoprotein (LDL), and triglyceride levels, thereby reducing the risk of hypertension, heart attack, and stroke. Recent research also suggests that EFAs may play a role in inhibiting the growth and spread of cancerous tumors.

There are two primary forms of essential fatty acids—omega-3 fatty acids and omega-6 fatty acids. Omega-3 fatty acids occur in three forms: alpha-linoleic acid (ALA), docosahexaenoic acid (DHA), and eicosapentaenoic acid (EPA). DHA and EPA are found in various cold-water fish, such as mackerel, salmon, and sardines, while ALA, which acts as a precursor to both DHA and EPA, is contained in fish oil and oils derived from flaxseeds, hemp, pumpkins, and walnuts. Flaxseeds, pumpkins, and walnuts by themselves are also good sources of omega-3 fatty acids. Since your body has to convert ALA into DHA and EPA, I recommend that people who are ill obtain omega-3 fatty acids from fish, as this spares the body from having to expend energy in the conversion process.

The primary forms of omega-6 fatty acids are gamma-linolenic acid (GLA) and linoleic acid. Both nutrients are found in black currant, borage seed, primrose, safflower, and sunflower oils, as well as fish oils. Almonds and pumpkin seeds are other good sources.

Ideally, it is best to obtain all your EFAs from the foods and oils mentioned above. But due to the importance of EFAs to health, supplementation is often advisable. EFA supplements are commonly available in capsule form. If you choose this option, make sure the capsules are fresh. To be certain, break a capsule open and smell it. If you notice a foul odor, toss it out. An easy way to meet your omega-3 EFA requirements is to take a capsule containing both EPA (300 milligrams) and DHA (200 milligrams) once a day. To ensure that you are receiving an adequate supply of omega-6 EFAs, take 1,000 milligrams of evening primrose oil a day.

Digestive Enzymes

Digestive enzymes are derived from plants and, as their name implies, are essential for proper digestion. These enzymes become active in the stomach, where they aid in the predigestion of food as it is consumed, enabling the body to more efficiently assimilate the foods' nutrients.

Increasingly, physicians and health practitioners are advising their clients and patients to use digestive enzyme supplements for better health. I also recommend that you consider supplementing with digestive enzymes at each of your meals. Doing so will not only help you better digest your meals and assimilate the nutrients they contain, but will also aid in your body's energy production. The enzymes I recommend are all plant-based, meaning that they are derived from raw fruits and vegetables. The primary plant-based enzymes are amylase, cellulase, disaccharidase, lipase, and protease.

Digestive enzymes are commonly packaged in combination so that their benefits can be maximized. For best results, take them at the start of each meal in the dosage recommended by the manufacturer. The following discussions will familiarize you with the digestive enzymes that are most important to your health.

Amylase

The digestive enzyme amylase is needed for the breakdown of long-chain carbohydrates, such as starches. As a result, amylase deficiencies—which can be caused by a lack of amylase from food sources as

---

Enzyme Deficiencies and Their Causes

All fruits and vegetables contain an abundant supply of enzymes, and in an ideal environment, you would derive all of the enzymes your body requires from the foods you eat. In today's world, however, even a diet high in fruits and vegetables may not provide you with all the enzymes your body needs. One reason for this is that enzymes are heat sensitive and are destroyed when the foods containing them are cooked in temperatures above 118°F. Microwaving also destroys enzymes. For this reason, it is best to eat fruits and vegetables raw or lightly steamed.

Numerous other factors can also cause enzyme deficiencies. Chief among them are commercial farming and food production methods, which use chemicals and pesticides; gene-splicing, genetic engineering, and hybridization; irradiation; and pasteurization, all of which deplete enzyme supplies in fruit and vegetable crops. Canning destroys enzymes, as well.

According to noted enzyme expert Lita Lee, PhD, author of *The Enzyme Cure,* other factors that can cause enzyme deficiencies include a high intake of unsaturated and hydrogenated fats, the consumption of fluoridated water, and exposure to radiation and electromagnetic fields, such as those emitted by computers and television screens. People who have mercury amalgam dental fillings and/or root canals can also suffer from enzyme deficiencies, according to Dr. Lee. Heavy metal toxicity, a condition that is far more widespread than most people realize, depletes enzyme activity, as well. For all of these reasons, supplementing with digestive enzymes is a good idea.

well as excess sugar consumption—can result in the incomplete digestion of carbohydrates.

Like other enzymes, amylase performs more than one function in the body. In addition to carbohydrate digestion, amylase helps ease muscle soreness following physical exertion, and can help relieve stiff joints and conditions such as writer's cramp. It also helps to prevent and eliminate the buildup of dead white blood cells known as leukocytes. Moreover, according to Dr. Lee, amylase is helpful in preventing and managing allergic reactions; canker sores; fungal infections; gallbladder and liver problems; herpes; hives; lung conditions such as asthma and bronchitis; and skin rash.

Cellulase

Cellulase is essential for the proper digestion of fiber, which it helps convert into usable glucose for energy. Since no enzyme similar to cellulase is manufactured by the body, it is vital to eat cellulase-rich foods. The best food sources are raw fruits, raw vegetables, and whole grains.

Besides helping to digest fiber, cellulase also digests yeast and fungi, making it useful in the prevention and relief of candidiasis (systemic yeast infection), as well as bowel and vaginal yeast infections. Cellulase also helps digest certain neurotoxins related to facial pain and paralysis, is effective in neutralizing intestinal bloating and flatulence, and can help stop acute food allergies.

Disaccharidase

Disaccharidase plays a vital role in the digestion of sugars known as disaccharides. The three primary forms of disaccharides are lactose (milk sugar), maltose (grain sugar), and sucrose (cane sugar). Disaccharidase breaks these sugars down into glucose and fructose, which the body can then use. The consumption of refined sugar—a staple of the standard American diet—is the primary cause of disaccharidase deficiency.

According to Dr. Lee, disaccharidase can be helpful in relieving the physical and mental/emotional symptoms caused by sugar intolerance. Physical symptoms of sugar intolerance include dizziness, gastrointestinal conditions, and respiratory problems, particularly asthma. Mental/emotional symptoms include anxiety and depression, attention deficit disorder (ADD), bipolar disorders, hyperactivity, mood swings, and panic attacks. Disaccharidase can also help mitigate symptoms associated with lactose intolerance, such as constipation and diarrhea, and can help reverse the spread of candidiasis.

Lipase

The enzyme lipase helps the body digest fats, primarily triglycerides. In addition, lipase enzymes play an integral role in maintaining cell wall permeability, which allows nutrients to easily pass into your body's cells, and permits cellular wastes to pass out of the cells for elimination.

Lipase deficiency is fairly common, and occurs primarily in people who have an intolerance to fats and people who are intolerant to complex carbohydrates. Such people have a higher risk of developing atherosclerosis and other cardiovascular problems, chronic fatigue, diabetes, gallbladder problems, high cholesterol, hypertension, and varicose veins. They are also more likely to suffer from weight gain and obesity, and more apt to suffer from deficiencies of fat-soluble vitamins, such as vitamins A, D, and E.

Protease

The enzyme protease breaks proteins down into amino acids, which are essential for the growth, maintenance, and repair of your body's tissues. This enzyme is also required for energy production and optimal mental function, as well as many other physiological processes. Protease also digests the protein coating of bacteria, viruses, and other microorganisms, making them better able to be identified and eliminated by the immune system. Finally, protease protects against blood clots, and can help eliminate them should they form.

When protease is lacking in the diet, incompletely digested proteins can result in low blood sugar (hypoglycemia), and in an overly alkaline pH in the bloodstream. This, in turn, forces the kidneys to work overtime to excrete alkaline reserves into the urine. According to Dr. Lee, the buildup of excess alkaline reserves can often result in a state of anxiety.

MSM

MSM (methyl sulfonyl methane) is a sulfur compound that naturally occurs in the body. When available in adequate amounts, it helps the body build healthy cells and enhances the health and growth of hair, muscles, nails, and skin. It also plays an important role in the manufacture of collagen, the primary component of cartilage and connective tissue.

In recent years, MSM has gained a reputation as a natural means of alleviating the pain of arthritis. Arthritis patients who take MSM supplements have experienced significant improvement in their symptoms. But MSM's benefits are not limited to arthritis pain. Additional research indicates that this compound can increase hair and nail growth and help repair damaged skin. It also enhances the ability of body fluids to more easily pass through tissues, thus improving the delivery of oxygen and nutrients to the cells, as well as the elimination of cellular waste products.

Although MSM is found in fresh fruits and vegetables, meat, milk, and seafood, most people are deficient in sulfur because of the body's continued use and excretion of the substance. This deficiency is made worse by the fact that most diets lack adequate amounts of MSM-rich foods. Moreover, levels of the compound are often lacking in foods due to commercial food harvesting, processing, and packaging methods. MSM levels in the body also naturally decline with age, leading to a greater risk of fatigue, organ and tissue malfunction, and susceptibility to disease.

MSM is an extremely safe and nontoxic substance, very similar to water in that it is almost impossible to consume too much of it. The body uses what it needs and eliminates the rest. I recommend that you supplement with 2,000 to 10,000 milligrams of MSM daily, depending on your specific nutritional needs. For best results, take the supplement with meals.

GREEN DRINKS

By now, you understand why I recommend that you eat plenty of fresh dark green leafy vegetables throughout the day. More than any other food group, vegetables—green and otherwise—provide you with the most alkalizing benefits, along with many essential vitamins, minerals, and enzymes. When these foods are eaten in sufficient quantities, they can significantly reduce the toxic effects of acid buildup. But I also realize that it is not always easy to follow this recommendation. Many of us have fast-paced lives that can make it difficult to find the time needed to prepare and eat optimally healthy meals. That's why I am a big proponent of green drinks.

For those of you who may not be familiar with green drinks, allow me to give you a little background on these highly nutritious foods. Green drink products are a relatively new type of supplement that provides a wide array of vital vitamins, minerals, enzymes, and other nutrients in a concentrated green powder that can be mixed with fresh-squeezed juice or pure filtered water. There are a variety of green drink products on the market, including single-ingredient powders made from wheatgrass, barley grass, or algae. Single drinks are acceptable, but I prefer multi-ingredient formulas that contain an abundant mixture of grasses, sprouts, and green and colored vegetables—broccoli, beets, cabbage, celery, and kale, for instance—along with herbs such as parsley, garlic, and ginger, which can boost the energy power of the product. Formulas that also contain MSM are even better, since this sulfur-rich compound acts synergistically with the other ingredients to enhance their bioavailability, making them easier for your body to use.

Besides green drinks' ability to enhance your body's internal pH level, as well as the wealth of nutrients they offer, a single glass is the equivalent of five to seven servings of vegetables. Moreover, because the nutrients found in green drinks are predigested, your body can make use of them immediately, putting them to work to restore the body's acid-alkaline balance.

Green drinks also contain abundant amounts of chlorophyll. As discussed in Chapter 5, chlorophyll is nearly identical in molecular structure to your blood's hemoglobin. As a result, this substance provides the core nutrients necessary to feed and maintain your body's hemoglobin supply, and can be a powerful aid in regenerating your body at the cellular level. It also acts as a potent cleanser, detoxifier, and immune enhancer, and boosts red blood cell count, which in turn increases your body's ability to utilize oxygen. In nature, the two most abundant sources of chlorophyll are wheatgrass and barley grass, which is why you should be certain that the green drink product you choose contains both of these foods.

A glass of green drink is a wonderful way to start the day, as it will supply you with many of your nutritional requirements. For even better results, add the mixture to a bottle of water and drink it throughout the day. Because of the concentration of alkalizing nutrients, I often recommend green drinks to clients who need an extra boost to recover from over-acidity. Usually such people start to notice significant improvements in their health in a matter of weeks, as long as they also follow the basic eating and supplement principles discussed here and in Chapter 5.

Guidelines for Using Nutritional Supplements

By choosing good-quality nutritional supplements and using them wisely, you'll help your body recover from over-acidity and provide it with the nutrients it needs to function properly. The following guidelines will help you get the most out of your supplements.

❑ Unless otherwise indicated, take nutritional supplements with meals. This will aid in their absorption, making it easier for your body to derive the benefits such supplements can provide.

❑ To enhance their effectiveness, take fat-soluble nutrients—vitamins A and E, beta-carotene, and essential fatty acids (EFAs)—with the meal of the day that has the highest fat content.

❑ Get your physician's approval before taking high doses of any nutritional supplement. Also be sure to divide the doses up so that you take them throughout the day, rather than all at once. This will make it easier for your body to make use of them.

❑ Avoid taking mineral supplements with high-fiber meals, as fiber can interfere with your body's ability to absorb minerals.

❑ When supplementing with individual B vitamins, also supplement with a complete vitamin B-complex supplement, as B vitamins work most effectively in concert with one another.

❑ Avoid supplements that contain artificial sweeteners, binders, coatings, fillers, fructose, or preservatives.

❑ If you are using prescribed medications, be sure to inform your physician about your nutritional supplement use, as certain nutrients and herbs can interfere with the action of some drugs, and may even cause adverse side effects.

Tips for Using Green Drink Supplements

The following guidelines will help you most effectively use green drink products to improve and maintain your health.

❏ Select a product that contains a wide range of organically grown and processed vegetables, sprouts, grasses, and herbs, rather than a single-ingredient formula. For added benefits, choose a product that contains MSM.

❏ Avoid products that contain caffeine, corn, eggs, dairy products, gluten or other wheat byproducts (wheatgrass is gluten-free), processed starches and sugars, yeast, or artificial colors, flavors, or fragrances.

❏ Always use pure filtered water when preparing your green drinks.

❏ Drink your green drink at least fifteen to thirty minutes before or after meals. This will allow your body to more easily assimilate the nutrients provided by the drink.

❏ For optimal results, have a green drink in the morning prior to breakfast. For an added boost, drink another glass or two later in the day as well.

CONCLUSION

While no amount of nutritional supplementation can replace a healthy diet, there is no question that the supplements discussed above are important. This is especially true if you are struggling with over-acidity and the health problems associated with that condition. By eating well and supplementing wisely, and by following the general health recommendations covered in Chapter 2, you can make steady and significant progress in your journey to vibrant health.

Now that you understand all of the self-care principles involved in restoring your body's acid-alkaline balance, it is time for you to start putting them into action. To help jump-start the process, I've created a fourteen-day food plan that is easy to follow, and provides a diet that is both delicious and rich in nutrients. Turn the page, and Chapter 7 will start you on the road to health.

7

The 14-Day Diet and Sample Recipes

When I work with first-time clients who want to improve their health and optimize their acid-alkaline balance, I recommend that they begin by following a two-week cleansing diet, which they can then repeat every three or four months. This diet introduces them to meals that are 80-percent alkaline and 20-percent acidic. When clients suffer from serious acidity, I encourage them to follow the vegetarian version of the diet, which is 100-percent alkalizing and provides even faster results. Having worked with many clients over the years, I have found that this 14-Day Diet quickly and safely increases vitality and well-being. The very same dietary suggestions and recipes that I share with my clients constitute the rest of this chapter, so that you, too, can start to improve your health.

BEFORE YOU BEGIN

The two versions of the 14-Day Diet, which begin on page 130, tell you exactly what to eat for each and every meal of the day. This makes it easy to get the foods you need to regain your health, and to avoid the foods that may be compromising your well-being. But to get maximum benefits from the 14-Day Diet, it's important to understand some basics, to get yourself in the right frame of mind, and to make a commitment to a healthy new way of eating. The following guidelines should get you started.

Avoid Fruit

As you read the meal suggestions that follow, you will notice that none of them includes fruit—other than lemon juice mixed with water. The reason for this is simple. During this cleansing phase, you want to give your body the opportunity to rid itself not only of toxic acids, but also of any harmful microorganisms and cellular waste products that might be present. This includes *Candida albicans*, a type of yeast that can cause candidiasis (systemic yeast overgrowth). Like other yeasts, *Candida albicans* feeds upon sugar. Since all fruits contain fructose, a naturally occurring sugar, for the first two weeks of your move towards a healthier diet, I recommend that fruits and most fruit juices be avoided. After those two weeks, you can begin to reintroduce fruit into your diet. Just remember to do so sparingly, and to eat fruit on its own rather than combining it with other foods.

Know When to Stop

The serving sizes of the recipes that begin on page 140 are simply guidelines. If you find that you need to eat larger portions in order to feel satisfied, by all means do so. As a general rule, however, try to walk away from each meal feeling only 75 to 85 percent full, so that your body can more easily digest and assimilate the foods you consume. Because of the interval between the time we consume food and the time we feel satisfied, many of us overeat without realizing it. If you can learn to stop eating before you feel full, you will allow your appetite to catch up to your brain.

Understand Your Own Eating Habits

To mentally prepare yourself for a healthier way of eating, consider when and why you eat. Often, we eat not because we are hungry, but simply out of habit, boredom, or loneliness, or for comfort. Under such circumstances, food serves as a substitute for something else—for resolution of an emotional issue, perhaps. By becoming more conscious of your eating habits, you will soon begin to know when you are truly hungry, and when you are eating out of habit or as a means of making yourself feel better. Try to discipline yourself to eat only when you are hungry.

Eat Three Meals Daily

I strongly recommend that you eat three meals a day, not only during the 14-Day Diet phase, but at all times. It is especially important that you do not skip breakfast, as it supplies you with the fuel you need to start your day productively and full of energy. Also, try to eat your last meal no later than 8:00 PM so that your body is not forced to cope with digestion after you retire to bed.

Prepare Healthy Snacks in Advance

Between meals, you may find yourself wishing for a snack. You are the best judge of when you need a bite to eat, so prepare your healthy snacks in advance. You can choose a few pieces of celery or carrots, half a cup of plain nonfat yogurt (ideally organic), some fresh almonds, or brown rice cakes with almond or cashew butter. After the first two weeks, you can also snack on a piece of fruit.

Choose the Meal Plan That Best Suits You

As mentioned earlier, this chapter provides two versions of the 14-Day Diet—one for nonvegetarians and one for vegetarians. Because the vegetarian plan is 100-percent alkalizing, I encourage nonvegetarians to eat vegetarian meals from time to time for the cleansing benefits they provide. If you cannot find one or more of the ingredients called for in the meal plans, feel free to substitute healthy alternatives. Additionally, if you follow a vegan diet—if you avoid eggs, milk, and all other dairy products—feel free to substitute tofu or egg substitute. Finally, please be sure to drink plenty of pure filtered water, not only during the two weeks of the diet, but all the time, to ensure that your body is properly hydrated.

Find the Right Food

Some of the foods on my diet plan—spelt pasta, for instance—may be unfamiliar to you. If that is the case, I suggest you learn a little about these foods by buying and using them *before* you go on the plan. Most supermarkets now have health food sections, and most towns have health food stores, so start exploring. The more you shop in the appropriate markets, and the more familiar you become with any new foods, the more comfortable you will be in adding these items to your diet.

Dump the Junk

Carefully examine your pantry and your refrigerator. How much of the food that's now in your house is truly unhealthy for you? If you're like most people, you'll find ice cream, cookies, candy, and sugary snacks—

lots of make-believe foods that can provide you with comfort, but that offer absolutely no health value. If you truly intend to follow the 14-Day Diet, I suggest you rid your home of all those temptations that are right in front of you. Give them to a food bank, share them with your friends or coworkers, or simply throw them out. Then replace the junk food with real food that will enhance your health and well-being.

Make the Commitment

The next time you visit the local shopping mall, or even take a walk through your own neighborhood, look carefully at the people around you. As a nation, too many of us are obese. Now consider the future of all those overweight people. Is it a future filled with health and vitality, or is it one of fatigue and ill health? If you want to regain control of your own health, you must promise yourself to see the program through to its completion.

Foods to Avoid

The following foods, as well as all products that contain them, should be avoided at all times—not just during the 14-Day Diet. Why? All of these foods are known to create acid-alkaline imbalances.

Sugar

Avoid sugar and all quick-acting carbohydrates, including sucrose, fructose, maltose, lactose, glycogen, glucose, sorbitol, galactose, monosaccharides, and polysaccharides. Also avoid honey, molasses, maple syrup, and other high-sugar products.

Yeast, Breads, and Pastries

Stay away from baked goods—including breads, rolls, cakes, and pastries—that are made with yeast. Also avoid the yeast-extract spreads Marmite, Vegemite, and Promite. Finally, steer clear of nutritional supplements made with yeast. (When buying supplements, look for the words "Yeast Free" on the label.)

Alcoholic Beverages

During the 14-Day Diet, avoid all alcoholic beverages. Once you have completed the diet and are experiencing improved levels of health and vitality, it is permissible to have a glass of wine from time to time. I recommend red wine because of its health benefits. But whenever you drink wine, be sure to increase your water intake afterwards, because all alcohol is dehydrating.

Condiments, Sauces, and Vinegar

Avoid eating mustard, tomato sauce, Worcestershire sauce, soy sauce, pickles, horseradish, mince, tamari, and miso. Avoid vinegar of all kinds, as well as foods that contain vinegar, such as salad dressings. Freshly squeezed lemon juice may be substituted. You may also use sea or Celtic salt, herbs, and pepper—either black or red—to add flavor to your meals.

Processed and Smoked Meats

Avoid pickled and smoked meats, including sausages, hot dogs, corned beef, bacon, and ham. Such meats often contain chemical additives that are not healthy. Moreover, the process of pickling and curing (smoking) meat makes it more difficult to digest.

Leftovers

Unless leftovers have been promptly and properly refrigerated, throw them out. Mold can quickly grow on leftover food. As far as possible, prepare only what you intend to eat at one sitting so that little or no food will remain at the end of the meal.

Fruit Juices

Avoid drinking canned, bottled, and frozen juices, including orange, grape, and apple juice.

Coffee and Tea

Avoid coffee—both regular and decaffeinated—and standard teas. A healthier option is herbal teas.

Cheeses and Other Dairy Products

Avoid all cheeses, as well as snacks that contain cheese. Also avoid milk, buttermilk, sour cream, and sour milk products.

Nuts

Except Brazil nuts and almonds, all nuts should be avoided. Especially avoid peanuts and pistachios, as these products commonly contain mold.

Fourteen days may not seem like a long time, but to some, it can feel like a year. Understand that this is the first step towards better health, and be ready to experience the good changes that will take place. Take your calendar, circle the date that you will begin the program, and look forward to the benefits that are yours for the taking—weight loss, better skin, abundant energy, and best of all, good health.

THE 14-DAY DIET FOR NONVEGETARIANS

The following menu, designed for nonvegetarians, will guide you through your 14-Day Diet. Please note that whenever a specific dish is recommended, it is followed by the number of the page on which you can find the appropriate recipe. All of the recipes are presented at the end of this chapter, and should serve as a springboard to a healthier way of cooking and eating.

You will note that every meal begins with either a glass of pure water and fresh lemon juice, or a green drink. As indicated, either drink should be consumed fifteen minutes before you actually sit down to eat your meal, as this will prevent the beverage from interfering with the digestive process. When mixing up the green drink, you'll want to use eight ounces of pure water plus the amount of green drink powder specified by the manufacturer. To make water with lemon juice, add the freshly squeezed juice of one organically grown lemon to an eight-ounce glass of pure water.

Although this menu does not recommend specific snacks, as discussed on page 127, snacks are allowable as long as you stick to those foods included on the diet—raw vegetables or a half cup of plain nonfat organic yogurt, for instance. During this two-week period, you should avoid snacking on fruit, as fruit contains natural sugar that can inhibit the cleansing process.

DAY 1
Breakfast	Green drink (15 minutes before eating) ½ to 1 cup cooked oat bran with almond milk
Lunch	Water with lemon juice (15 minutes before eating) 1 serving Tuna-Stuffed Avocado (see page 147) 1 cup green salad with lemon juice dressing 1 rice cake

Dinner	Water with lemon juice or green drink (15 minutes before eating)
	1 serving Vegetable Soup (see page 143)
	1 cup wild and brown rice with almonds
	1/2 to 1 cup steamed green beans

DAY 2

Breakfast	Green drink (15 minutes before eating)
	1 to 2 pieces Fiesta Toast (see page 144)
Lunch	Water with lemon juice (15 minutes before eating)
	1 serving Curried Chicken Salad (see page 148)
	1 serving Red Lettuce and Radish Sprout Salad (see page 148)
	1 rice cake
Dinner	Water with lemon juice or green drink (15 minutes before eating)
	1 serving Orange Roughy With Butter Sauce and Almonds (see page 149)
	1 cup brown rice
	1/2 to 1 cup steamed vegetables

DAY 3

Breakfast	Green drink (15 minutes before eating)
	1 serving Breakfast Olé (see page 140)
Lunch	Water with lemon juice (15 minutes before eating)
	1 serving Spinach and Egg Salad (see page 146)
	3 ounces white albacore tuna
	1 rice cake
Dinner	Water with lemon juice or green drink (15 minutes before eating)
	4 ounces baked turkey breast
	1 serving Roasted Potatoes (see page 156)
	1 cup green salad with lemon juice dressing

DAY 4

Breakfast	Green drink (15 minutes before eating)
	1 cup puffed brown rice cereal with almond milk
Lunch	Water with lemon juice (15 minutes before eating)
	1 cup spelt pasta with Pesto Latino (see page 159)
	1 cup green salad with lemon juice dressing
Dinner	Water with lemon juice or green drink (15 minutes before eating)
	1 serving Garlic Chicken (see page 150)
	1 serving Spinach and Egg Salad (see page 146)
	1/2 to 1 cup steamed vegetables

DAY 5

Breakfast	Green drink (15 minutes before eating) 2 scrambled eggs 2 slices turkey bacon 1 piece Fiesta Toast (see page 144)
Lunch	Water with lemon juice (15 minutes before eating) 1 serving Chicken Salad (see page 147) 1 rice cake
Dinner	Water with lemon juice or green drink (15 minutes before eating) 1 cup brown rice with black beans ½ to 1 cup steamed vegetables 1 cup green salad with lemon juice dressing

DAY 6

Breakfast	Green drink (15 minutes before eating) 1 serving Vegetable Omelet (see page 140)
Lunch	Water with lemon juice (15 minutes before eating) 4 ounces roasted chicken breast 1 cup green salad with lemon juice dressing 1 rice cake
Dinner	Water with lemon juice or green drink (15 minutes before eating) 1 serving Orange Roughy With Butter Sauce and Almonds (see page 149) ½ to 1 cup steamed vegetables 1 cup green salad with lemon juice dressing

DAY 7

Breakfast	Green drink (15 minutes before eating) 1 serving Breakfast Burrito (see page 142)
Lunch	Water with lemon juice (15 minutes before eating) Turkey sandwich on yeast-free bread 1 rice cake
Dinner	Water with lemon juice or green drink (15 minutes before eating) 4 ounces roasted chicken breast 1 cup brown rice 1 serving Spinach and Egg Salad (see page 146) ½ avocado

DAY 8

Breakfast	Green drink (15 minutes before eating) 1 cup plain nonfat organic yogurt Oat Bran Muffin (see page 141)
Lunch	Water with lemon juice (15 minutes before eating) 1 serving Tuna-Stuffed Avocado (see page 147) 1 cup green salad with lemon juice dressing 1 rice cake
Dinner	Water with lemon juice or green drink (15 minutes before eating) 1 serving Mediterranean Moussaka (see page 154) ½ to 1 cup steamed asparagus 1 cup green salad with lemon juice dressing

DAY 9

Breakfast	Green drink (15 minutes before eating) 1 serving Vegetable Soup (see page 143) 1 to 2 pieces yeast-free toast
Lunch	Water with lemon juice (15 minutes before eating) Turkey sandwich on yeast-free bread 1 cup green salad with lemon juice dressing
Dinner	Water with lemon juice or green drink (15 minutes before eating) 1 serving Italian Soup (see page 144) 1 cup spinach salad with lemon juice dressing 1 rice cake

DAY 10

Breakfast	Green drink (15 minutes before eating) 1 poached egg 1 to 2 pieces yeast-free toast
Lunch	Water with lemon juice (15 minutes before eating) 4 ounces roasted chicken breast 1 cup green salad with lemon juice dressing
Dinner	Water with lemon juice or green drink (15 minutes before eating) 4 ounces roast turkey tenders ½ to 1 cup steamed vegetables ½ cup brown rice 1 serving Spinach and Egg Salad (see page 146)

Day 11

Breakfast	Green drink (15 minutes before eating) 1 serving Breakfast Burrito (see page 142)
Lunch	Water with lemon juice (15 minutes before eating) 4 ounces baked chicken breast $\frac{1}{2}$ to 1 cup steamed zucchini Sliced tomatoes
Dinner	Water with lemon juice or green drink (15 minutes before eating) 1 serving Roasted Potatoes (see page 156) 1 cup brown rice 1 cup green salad with lemon juice dressing $\frac{1}{2}$ to 1 cup steamed green beans

Day 12

Breakfast	Green drink (15 minutes before eating) $\frac{1}{2}$ to 1 cup cooked oat bran with almond milk
Lunch	Water with lemon juice (15 minutes before eating) 1 serving Curried Chicken Salad (see page 148) 1 rice cake
Dinner	Water with lemon juice or green drink (15 minutes before eating) 1 serving Pasta Primavera (page 156) 1 cup green salad with lemon juice dressing

Day 13

Breakfast	Green drink (15 minutes before eating) 1 serving Breakfast Olé (see page 140)
Lunch	Water with lemon juice (15 minutes before eating) 1 serving Tuna-Stuffed Avocado (see page 147) 1 cup green salad with lemon juice dressing 1 rice cake
Dinner	Water with lemon juice or green drink (15 minutes before eating) 1 cup spelt spaghetti with marinara sauce 1 cup green salad with lemon juice dressing $\frac{1}{2}$ to 1 cup steamed vegetables

Day 14

Breakfast	Green drink (15 minutes before eating) 1 serving Vegetable Soup (see page 143) 1 to 2 pieces yeast-free toast

Lunch	Water with lemon juice (15 minutes before eating) 1 serving Marinated Buckwheat Salad (see page 158) 1 rice cake
Dinner	Water with lemon juice or green drink (15 minutes before eating) 4 ounces broiled salmon 1 cup brown rice 1 cup green salad with lemon juice dressing 1/2 to 1 cup steamed vegetables

THE 14-DAY DIET FOR VEGETARIANS

The following menu, designed for vegetarians, will guide you through your 14-Day Diet. Just like the menu presented on pages 130 to 135, whenever a specific dish is recommended, it is followed by the number of the page on which you can find the appropriate recipe. All of the recipes are presented at the end of this chapter.

Again, every meal begins with either a glass of pure water and fresh lemon juice, or a green drink, either of which should be consumed fifteen minutes before you actually sit down to eat your meal, as this will prevent the beverage from interfering with the digestive process.

Like the nonvegetarian diet, this one does not recommend specific snacks. Snacks are allowable, though. Just be sure to stick to the foods discussed on page 127.

DAY 1	
Breakfast	Green drink (15 minutes before eating) 1/2 cup to 1 cup cooked oat bran with almond milk
Lunch	Water with lemon juice (15 minutes before eating) Stir-fried veggie wrap with tofu 1 cup green salad with lemon juice dressing 1 rice cake
Dinner	Water with lemon juice or green drink (15 minutes before eating) 1 serving Vegetable Soup (see page 143) 1 cup wild and brown rice with almonds 1/2 to 1 cup steamed green beans

DAY 2

Breakfast	Green drink (15 minutes before eating) 1 to 2 pieces Fiesta Toast (see page 144)
Lunch	Water with lemon juice (15 minutes before eating) 1 cup veggie pasta with white beans 1 serving Red Lettuce and Radish Sprout Salad (see page 148) 1 rice cake
Dinner	Water with lemon juice or green drink (15 minutes before eating) 1 serving Mediterranean Moussaka (see page 154) $\frac{1}{2}$ to 1 cup steamed vegetables 1 cup green salad with lemon juice dressing

DAY 3

Breakfast	Green drink (15 minutes before eating) 1 serving Breakfast Olé (see page 140)
Lunch	Water with lemon juice (15 minutes before eating) 1 serving Spinach and Egg Salad (see page 146) 4 ounces grilled or roasted tofu 1 rice cake
Dinner	Water with lemon juice or green drink (15 minutes before eating) 1 serving Green Lentils With Garlic and Cilantro (see page 157) $\frac{1}{2}$ to 1 cup steamed broccoli 1 cup green salad with lemon juice dressing

DAY 4

Breakfast	Green drink (15 minutes before eating) 1 cup puffed brown rice cereal with almond milk
Lunch	Water with lemon juice (15 minutes before eating) 1 cup spelt pasta with Pesto Latino (see page 159) 1 cup green salad with lemon juice dressing 1 rice cake
Dinner	Water with lemon juice or green drink (15 minutes before eating) 1 serving Italian Soup (see page 144) 1 serving Spinach and Egg Salad (see page 146) $\frac{1}{2}$ to 1 cup steamed vegetables

DAY 5

Breakfast	Green drink (15 minutes before eating) 1 serving Vegetable Omelet (see page 140)

Lunch	Water with lemon juice (15 minutes before eating)
	1 cup brown rice with black beans
	1/2 to 1 cup steamed vegetables

Dinner	Water with lemon juice or green drink (15 minutes before eating)
	1 serving Broccoli Ziti With Garlic (see page 155)
	1 cup green salad with lemon juice dressing
	1 rice cake

DAY 6

Breakfast	Green drink (15 minutes before eating)
	1 serving Vegetable Omelet (see page 140)

Lunch	Water with lemon juice (15 minutes before eating)
	1 serving Veggie Chili (see page 145)
	1 cup green salad with lemon juice dressing

Dinner	Water with lemon juice or green drink (15 minutes before eating)
	1 serving Blackened Tofu (see page 151)
	1/2 to 1 cup steamed vegetables
	1 cup green salad with lemon juice dressing

DAY 7

Breakfast	Green drink (15 minutes before eating)
	1 serving Breakfast Burrito (see page 142)

Lunch	Water with lemon juice (15 minutes before eating)
	Roasted veggie sandwich on yeast-free bread
	1 rice cake

Dinner	Water with lemon juice or green drink (15 minutes before eating)
	4 ounces baked eggplant with soy mozzarella
	1 cup spinach salad with lemon juice dressing
	1/2 avocado

DAY 8

Breakfast	Green drink (15 minutes before eating)
	1 cup plain nonfat organic yogurt
	Oat Bran Muffin (see page 141)

Lunch	Water with lemon juice (15 minutes before eating)
	1 cup spelt pasta with Pesto Latino (see page 159)
	1 cup green salad with lemon juice dressing
	1 rice cake

Dinner	Water with lemon juice or green drink (15 minutes before eating)
	1 serving Mediterranean Moussaka (see page 154)
	½ to 1 cup steamed asparagus
	1 cup green salad with lemon juice dressing

DAY 9

Breakfast	Green drink (15 minutes before eating)
	1 poached egg
	1 to 2 pieces yeast-free toast

Lunch	Water with lemon juice (15 minutes before eating)
	Stir-fried veggie wrap
	1 cup green salad with lemon juice dressing

Dinner	Water with lemon juice or green drink (15 minutes before eating)
	1 serving Green Lentils With Garlic and Cilantro (see page 157)
	1 serving Spinach and Egg Salad (see page 146)
	1 rice cake

DAY 10

Breakfast	Green drink (15 minutes before eating)
	1 serving Vegetable Soup (see page 143)
	1 to 2 pieces yeast-free bread

Lunch	Water with lemon juice (15 minutes before eating)
	Veggie burger on yeast-free bread
	1 cup green salad with lemon juice dressing

Dinner	Water with lemon juice or green drink (15 minutes before eating)
	1 serving Italian Soup (see page 144)
	1 cup spinach salad with lemon juice dressing
	1 rice cake

DAY 11

Breakfast	Green drink (15 minutes before eating)
	½ to 1 cup cooked oat bran with almond milk

Lunch	Water with lemon juice (15 minutes before eating)
	1 cup spelt pasta salad
	1 rice cake

Dinner	Water with lemon juice or green drink (15 minutes before eating)
	Veggie burger on yeast-free bread
	1 serving Vegetable Soup (see page 143)
	1 cup green salad with lemon juice dressing

Day 12

Breakfast   Green drink (15 minutes before eating)
1 serving Breakfast Burrito (see page 142)

Lunch   Water with lemon juice (15 minutes before eating)
1 serving Roasted Eggplant and Tofu (page 153)
1/2 to 1 cup steamed zucchini
Tomato slices

Dinner   Water with lemon juice or green drink (15 minutes before eating)
1 serving Roasted Potatoes (see page 156) with 1 cup brown rice
1 cup green salad with lemon juice dressing
1/2 to 1 cup steamed green beans

Day 13

Breakfast   Green drink (15 minutes before eating)
1 serving Breakfast Olé (see page 140)

Lunch   Water with lemon juice (15 minutes before eating)
1 serving Florentine-Stuffed Tomatoes (see page 152)
1 cup green salad with lemon juice dressing
1 rice cake

Dinner   Water with lemon juice or green drink (15 minutes before eating)
1 cup spelt spaghetti with marinara sauce
1 cup green salad with lemon juice dressing
1/2 to 1 cup steamed vegetables

Day 14

Breakfast   Green drink (15 minutes before eating)
1 serving Vegetable Soup (see page 143)
1 to 2 pieces yeast-free toast

Lunch   Water with lemon juice (15 minutes before eating)
1 serving Marinated Buckwheat Salad (see page 158)
1 rice cake

Dinner   Water with lemon juice or green drink (15 minutes before eating)
1 serving Blackened Tofu (see page 151) with brown rice
1 cup green salad with lemon juice dressing
1/2 to 1 cup steamed vegetables

RECIPES

BREAKFAST OLÉ

YIELD: 4 SERVINGS

4 cups cooked brown rice

2 cups spinach torn into bite-sized pieces

2 cups cooked black beans

1 avocado, cut into chunks

Fresh salsa

Bragg Liquid Aminos

Salt to taste

Cayenne or black pepper to taste (optional)

Soaked almonds (optional)

1. Divide the rice equally among 4 serving bowls.

2. Top each portion of the rice with some of the spinach, beans, avocado, and salsa. Then drizzle with Bragg Liquid Aminos and salt and pepper to taste. Top with the soaked almonds if desired, and serve.

VEGETABLE OMELET

YIELD: 2 SERVINGS

4 large eggs

1 large tomato, diced

1 medium avocado, diced

2 large scallions, coarsely chopped

1/4 cup sliced green or black olives

2 tablespoons clarified butter

1. Place the eggs in a medium-sized bowl, and beat with a rotary beater or electric mixer until foamy. Stir in all of the remaining ingredients except for the butter.

2. Place the butter in a large skillet over medium heat, moving the pan back and forth until the bottom and sides are coated. Add the egg mixture and cook until the sides and bottom are golden brown.

3. Reduce the heat to low. Turn half of the omelet over the other half, cover, and cook until the egg is set. Serve hot.

OAT BRAN MUFFINS

YIELD: 12 MUFFINS

1 cup oat bran cereal

1 cup brown rice flour

2 teaspoons baking powder

1 teaspoon ground cinnamon

$\frac{1}{2}$ teaspoon baking soda

$\frac{1}{2}$ cup plain yogurt

$\frac{1}{4}$ cup 100-percent pure vegetable glycerin

2 large eggs, beaten

2 tablespoons olive oil

2 teaspoons orange extract

$\frac{1}{2}$ teaspoon vanilla extract

$\frac{1}{4}$ cup chopped walnuts

1. Preheat the oven to 400°F. Line 12 muffin cups with paper baking cups, and set aside.

2. Mix all of the dry ingredients, except for the walnuts, in one bowl. Mix all of the wet ingredients in another bowl. Pour the wet ingredients into the dry ingredients and stir just until moistened. Fold in the walnuts.

3. Spoon the batter into the muffin cups, filling each cup $^2/_3$ full. Bake for 15 to 18 minutes, or until a toothpick comes out clean when inserted in the center of a muffin. Allow to cool before serving.

BREAKFAST BURRITO

YIELD: 2 SERVINGS

2 tablespoons olive oil

2 red potatoes cut into ¼-inch cubes

2 large sprouted wheat tortillas

2 tablespoons butter

4 eggs, beaten with 1 tablespoon water

½ cup grated soy cheese

1 Serrano chili pepper, finely chopped

2 scallions, including half of the greens, chopped

Chopped fresh cilantro

Turkey bacon, cooked (optional)

Fresh Salsa (optional) (see page 159)

1. Place the olive oil in a medium-sized nonstick skillet, and heat over medium-high heat. Add the potatoes, and sauté for 10 to 20 minutes, or until cooked through. Remove the potatoes to a dish, and cover to keep warm.

2. Place the tortillas, one on top of the other, in a large ungreased skillet. Cook over low heat until heated through.

3. Heat the butter in the skillet over medium heat until it sizzles. Add the eggs and cook, stirring constantly to scramble. When the eggs are nearly done, turn off the heat and stir in the cheese, chili, scallions, and cilantro.

4. Scoop the eggs into the warm tortillas, and add the reserved potatoes and the bacon, if desired. Top with the salsa, if desired, fold the tortilla over the filling, and serve.

Variation

If you don't eat eggs, fill the burritos with scrambled tofu instead of scrambled eggs.

VEGETABLE SOUP

YIELD: 8 SERVINGS

2 tablespoons olive oil

3 cloves garlic, chopped

I large onion, diced

3 stalks celery, diced

6 carrots, peeled and diced

4 cups water

4 cups vegetable broth

4 medium-sized white or red potatoes, diced

3 cups fresh green beans cut into I-inch pieces

3 medium zucchini, diced

1/2 cup chopped fresh parsley

Salt and black pepper to taste

1. Heat the oil in a large stockpot over medium heat. Add the garlic and cook for 1 minute. Add the onion and cook for 5 minutes. Do not allow to brown. Add the celery and carrots and cook for 5 minutes, stirring frequently.

2. Add the water, broth, potatoes, green beans, and zucchini to the pot, and bring to a boil. Lower the heat to a simmer and cook for about 20 minutes, or just until the potatoes are tender.

3. Stir the parsley, salt, and pepper into the pot, and serve.

Variations

As desired, add any of the following to the soup: cubed cooked chicken, corn, summer squash, tomatoes, or chopped cabbage.

FIESTA TOAST

YIELD: 2 SERVINGS

2 pieces yeast-free bread

4–6 slices soy or rice cheese

Fresh Salsa (see page 159)

Salt and black pepper to taste

1. Preheat the broiler.

2. Toast the bread in a toaster or under the broiler. Arrange the toast on a cookie sheet, place 2 to 3 slices of cheese on each piece, and place under the broiler until melted. Watch carefully to prevent burning.

3. Top the toast with salsa, season with salt and pepper to taste, and serve.

ITALIAN SOUP

YIELD: 6 SERVINGS

2 teaspoons olive oil

2 cloves garlic, finely chopped

14-ounce can chopped tomatoes, drained

1 large sprig fresh rosemary, or 1 $\frac{1}{2}$ teaspoons dried

28-ounce can vegetable broth

2 cups water

2 cans (19 ounces each) chickpeas, rinsed and drained

6 ounces spelt elbow noodles

$\frac{1}{2}$ teaspoon black pepper

1. Heat the oil in a large pot over medium heat. Add the garlic and cook, stirring, for 1 minute. Add the tomatoes and rosemary. (If using fresh rosemary, be sure to take the sprigs off the stalk and chop them.) Simmer for 5 minutes. Pour in the broth and water, and bring to a simmer.

2. In a small bowl, mash 1 cup of the chickpeas with a fork or potato masher. Stir the mashed chickpeas into the pot, along with the elbow noodles and pepper. Simmer, uncovered, for 5 to 12 minutes, or until the pasta is tender.

3. Stir in the remaining whole chickpeas and cook just until heated through. Serve.

VEGGIE CHILI

YIELD: 4 SERVINGS

1 tablespoon olive oil

1 medium onion, diced

2 cloves garlic, minced

1 red bell pepper, diced

1 green bell pepper, diced

1 celery stalk, diced

28-ounce can diced tomatoes, undrained

7-ounce can kidney beans, rinsed and drained

7-ounce can black beans, rinsed and drained

1–2 tablespoons chili powder

Salt and black pepper to taste

2 tablespoons chopped fresh cilantro

Fresh cilantro sprigs (garnish)

Diced avocados (garnish)

1. Heat the oil in a large pot over medium heat. Add the onion and garlic and sauté for 3 to 5 minutes, or until tender. Add the red and green pepper and celery, and sauté for another 3 minutes.

2. Add the tomatoes, beans, and chili powder to the pot, and simmer for 20 to 30 minutes. Add salt and pepper to taste.

3. Stir in the chopped cilantro right before serving, and garnish each bowl with a sprig of cilantro and some diced avocado.

SPINACH AND EGG SALAD

YIELD: 4 SERVINGS

Salad

8 ounces fresh spinach leaves

2 cups thinly sliced zucchini

1 medium yellow bell pepper, thinly sliced

1 medium red bell pepper, thinly sliced

8 cherry tomatoes, halved

1/4 cup sliced green or black olives (optional)

2 large hard boiled eggs, chopped

Dressing

2 tablespoons sesame oil

2 tablespoons chopped onion

1/2 cup chicken broth

2 tablespoons 100-percent pure vegetable glycerin

1 tablespoon fresh lemon juice

2 tablespoons chopped fresh tarragon

1/2 teaspoon dry mustard

1 tablespoon arrowroot

1/4 cup cold water

1. To make the salad, tear the spinach into bite-sized pieces and place in a large bowl. Arrange the zucchini over the spinach, and place the peppers at random over the zucchini. Sprinkle with the tomatoes and olives, and cover with the chopped eggs. Cover and chill for 30 minutes to an hour.

2. To make the dressing, place the sesame oil and onion in a small nonstick skillet, and cook over medium heat until the onion is tender. Add the chicken broth, glycerin, lemon juice, tarragon, and dry mustard, and bring to a boil. Then reduce the heat to a simmer.

3. Mix the arrowroot with the water, and pour the mixture into the dressing. Heat, stirring constantly, until thick.

4. Pour the dressing, hot or cold, over the salad and serve.

CHICKEN SALAD

YIELD: 2 SERVINGS

2 chicken breasts, cooked, skinned, and shredded

2 scallions, chopped

$\frac{1}{2}$ cup chopped celery

$\frac{1}{2}$ cup seeded and diced cucumber

$\frac{1}{2}$ cup slivered almonds

$\frac{1}{2}$ cup mayonnaise or soy-based mayonnaise substitute

$\frac{1}{4}$ cup chopped red bell pepper

$\frac{1}{4}$ teaspoon dried dill (optional)

Salt and black pepper to taste

1. Place all of the ingredients in a large bowl and mix together.

2. Cover and chill for 4 to 6 hours to allow the flavors to blend before serving.

TUNA-STUFFED AVOCADO

YIELD: 2 SERVINGS

2 large lettuce leaves

1 medium avocado, scrubbed, pitted, and halved

6-ounce can solid white albacore tuna, or 4 ounces fresh tuna, cooked

2 stalks celery, finely chopped

2 small scallions, finely chopped

$\frac{1}{4}$ cup slivered almonds

$\frac{1}{2}$ teaspoon chopped fresh dill

1 medium lemon, cut into wedges

1. Place 1 lettuce leaf on each of 2 serving plates. Top each with an avocado half and cover with plastic wrap. Set aside.

2. Combine the tuna, celery, scallions, almonds, and dill in a large bowl. Fill each avocado half with half of the mixture, garnish with the lemon wedges, and serve.

RED LETTUCE AND RADISH SPROUT SALAD

YIELD: 4 SERVINGS

I large shallot, finely chopped

1 ½ tablespoons fresh lemon juice

¼ teaspoon salt

3 tablespoons extra virgin olive oil

I tablespoon walnut oil

4 good handfuls red-leaf lettuce

Salt to taste

I cup red radish sprouts

1. Combine the shallot, lemon juice, and salt in a bowl, and let stand for 10 to 15 minutes. Whisk in the oils, and set aside.

2. Place the greens in a large bowl, add a few pinches of salt, and toss. Add the dressing, distribute the sprouts, and toss until the greens are evenly coated with the dressing. Serve.

CURRIED CHICKEN SALAD

YIELD: 4 SERVINGS

8 ounces cooked chicken breast, cubed

2 large hard boiled eggs, coarsely chopped

3 scallions, chopped (greens included)

I medium red bell pepper, coarsely chopped

¼ cup mayonnaise

Curry powder to taste

4 large lettuce leaves

¼ cup slivered almonds, lightly toasted

1. Place the chicken, eggs, scallions, red pepper, mayonnaise, and curry powder in a large bowl, and stir to mix well. Set aside.

2. Place 1 lettuce leaf on each of 4 individual serving plates. Arrange a quarter of the chicken salad over the lettuce, sprinkle with the almonds, and serve.

ORANGE ROUGHY WITH BUTTER SAUCE AND ALMONDS

YIELD: 4 SERVINGS

$\frac{1}{2}$ cup clarified butter

1 teaspoon chopped fresh basil

1 teaspoon chopped fresh oregano

Garlic powder to taste

4 orange roughy fillets (6–8 ounces each)

$\frac{1}{2}$ cup sliced almonds

1 medium lemon, cut into wedges (garnish)

Fresh parsley sprigs (garnish)

1. Preheat the oven to 350ºF.

2. Heat the butter in a small skillet, add the basil, oregano, and garlic powder, and immediately remove from the heat.

3. Dip both sides of each piece of fish into the butter sauce, and arrange the fish in a baking dish. Pour any remaining sauce over the fish and sprinkle with the almonds.

4. Bake for 20 minutes, or until the fish can be easily flaked with a fork. Garnish with the lemon and parsley and serve.

GARLIC CHICKEN

YIELD: 6 SERVINGS

1 tablespoon olive oil

4 pounds bone-in chicken parts, skinned

Salt and black pepper to taste

30 cloves garlic, unpeeled (3–4 heads)

1¾ cups chicken stock

4 sprigs fresh thyme, or ¼ teaspoon dried

1 sprig fresh rosemary, or ¼ teaspoon dried

Fresh parsley, chopped (garnish)

1. Preheat the oven to 350°F.

2. Place the oil in a heavy-bottomed, flame-proof casserole dish wide enough to accommodate the chicken in a single layer. (If you have no flame-proof casserole, sauté the chicken in a large skillet and transfer to a casserole for baking.) Place over medium-high heat, add the chicken, and season to taste with salt and pepper. Sauté for 5 minutes, turn, and cook for another 5 minutes. Remove the chicken from the dish.

3. Add the garlic to the casserole dish and sauté, stirring, for 3 to 5 minutes, or until the garlic begins to brown.

4. Spread the garlic cloves in a single layer over the bottom of the casserole dish, and arrange the chicken over the garlic. Add the chicken stock, thyme, and rosemary, and cover tightly with aluminum foil.

5. Bake for 45 minutes. Test the chicken for doneness by cutting with a knife. If not quite cooked through, bake for 15 additional minutes, or until done.

6. Open the garlic cloves and spread the roasted garlic over yeast-free toast to accompany the chicken. Garnish the chicken with the parsley before serving.

BLACKENED TOFU

YIELD: *4–6 SERVINGS*

2 blocks (I pound each) firm tofu

2 1/2 teaspoons salt

I tablespoon sweet paprika

I teaspoon onion powder

I teaspoon garlic powder

1/2–I teaspoon cayenne pepper

3/4 teaspoon white pepper

3/4 teaspoon black pepper

1/2 teaspoon dried thyme

1/2 teaspoon dried oregano

6–8 tablespoons butter, melted
(preferably clarified)

1. Cut the tofu into 1/2-inch-thick slabs and drain on paper towels for at least 30 minutes, preferably with a weight on top. The tofu needs to be very dry.

2. Mix all of the spices in a shallow dish. Place the butter in a second dish and brush each piece of tofu with the butter. Then dredge the tofu in the spice mixture, patting it firmly onto the tofu.

3. Heat a cast-iron skillet over high heat until it is white-hot, about 15 minutes. Pour a teaspoon of melted butter onto each piece of tofu, then place it butter side down on the hot skillet and step back. Wait 2 minutes, turn, and repeat on the second side. Transfer to a platter and keep warm until all of the tofu has been cooked. Serve hot.

FLORENTINE-STUFFED TOMATOES

YIELD: 6 SERVINGS

6 large tomatoes

2 tablespoons olive oil

I medium onion, finely chopped

I large clove garlic, minced

I pound fresh spinach, cooked until wilted,
drained, and squeezed dry

2 cups cooked brown rice

I tablespoon coarsely chopped fresh basil

$\frac{1}{2}$ teaspoon ground nutmeg

$\frac{1}{4}$ cup chopped almonds

1. Preheat the oven to 400ºF.

2. Cut the tops off the tomatoes and scoop out the pulp. Set the tomatoes aside, and chop the pulp. Set aside.

3. Place the oil in a large skillet over medium heat. Add the onion and garlic, and sauté until tender. Add the spinach, tomato pulp, rice, basil, and nutmeg, and stir until the spinach and tomato are well coated with the seasonings. Remove from the heat.

4. Arrange the tomatoes in a buttered 8-inch baking dish. Divide the spinach filling among the tomatoes, top with the almonds, and bake for 15 to 20 minutes. Serve hot.

ROASTED EGGPLANT AND TOFU

YIELD: 2 SERVINGS

10-ounce block extra-firm tofu

2 tablespoons olive oil

2 cloves garlic, minced

1 eggplant, cut into 1/2-inch slices

Salt and black pepper to taste

Marinade

1/4 cup olive oil

2–4 tablespoons fresh lemon juice

2 tablespoons Bragg Liquid Aminos

1 clove garlic, minced

1. Cut the tofu into 1/2-inch-thick slabs and drain on paper towels for at least 30 minutes, preferably with a weight on top. The tofu needs to be very dry.

2. While the tofu is draining, place all of the marinade ingredients in a shallow bowl and stir to mix well. Place the drained tofu slices in the marinade, cover, and refrigerate for 4 to 6 hours or overnight, turning occasionally so that the tofu soaks up the flavors of the mixture.

3. Preheat the oven broiler.

4. Mix the olive oil and garlic together, and brush the eggplant with the oil. Sprinkle with the salt and pepper.

5. Remove the tofu from the marinade, discarding the marinade, and arrange the tofu and the eggplant in a broiler-safe baking dish. Broil for 4 to 5 minutes or until brown, turn, and repeat on the other side. Serve hot.

MEDITERRANEAN MOUSSAKA

YIELD: 8 SERVINGS

2 cups vegetable or chicken stock

³/₄ cup brown rice

2 medium eggplants, cut into ¹/₂-inch slices

3 tablespoons olive oil, divided

¹/₄ cup pine nuts

I large onion, diced

4 cloves garlic, minced

I teaspoon salt

¹/₂ teaspoon ground cumin

¹/₄ teaspoon ground allspice

¹/₄ teaspoon ground cardamom

Black pepper to taste

14¹/₂-ounce can crushed tomatoes

¹/₄ cup sliced kalamata olives

2 teaspoons fresh lemon juice

1. Preheat the oven to 375°.

2. Place the stock in a medium-sized saucepan, and bring to a boil over high heat. Stir in the rice, reduce the heat to medium-low, cover, and cook for about 20 minutes, or until all of the liquid has been absorbed. Set aside.

3. Arrange the eggplant slices on a baking sheet that has been lightly coated with cooking spray or oil, and brush the tops of the slices with 2 tablespoons of the olive oil. Bake for about 20 minutes, or until softened and lightly browned. Set aside.

4. Place the remaining tablespoon of olive oil in a medium-sized skillet and add the pine nuts. Cook over medium-low heat, stirring constantly, until golden brown. Add the onion, garlic, salt, cumin, allspice, cardamom, and pepper, and sauté for about 5 minutes, or until tender.

5. Stir the tomatoes, olives, and lemon juice into the onion mixture, and cook for 2 minutes.

6. Reduce the oven temperature to 350°F. Lightly coat a 9-x-13-inch baking dish with cooking spray or oil. Arrange in layers half of the rice, half of the eggplant slices, and half of the sauce. Repeat the layers.

7. Cover and bake for 30 to 40 minutes, or until bubbly. Serve hot.

BROCCOLI ZITI WITH GARLIC

YIELD: 4 SERVINGS

10- or 12-ounce package spelt ziti

$^1/_3$ cup soymilk

4 cups broccoli florets

$^1/_4$ cup olive oil

4 cloves garlic, minced

Crushed red pepper flakes to taste

$^1/_3$ cup grated soy Parmesan cheese

Salt and pepper to taste

1. Prepare the pasta according to package directions. Drain, return to the pot, and toss with the soymilk. Remove from the heat, cover, and set aside.

2. Steam the broccoli until bright green but still crisp. Set aside.

3. Heat the oil in a small skillet over low heat. Add the garlic and red pepper flakes, and cook for 1 to 2 minutes.

4. Add the steamed broccoli and garlic mixture to the pasta, and stir to mix. Stir in the soy cheese and salt and pepper to taste, and serve.

PASTA PRIMAVERA

YIELD: 2 SERVINGS

8-ounce package spelt noodles

2 tablespoons olive oil

2 cloves garlic, minced

2 zucchini, julienned

2 carrots, peeled and julienned

I cup fresh or frozen (thawed) peas

$\frac{1}{2}$ cup thinly sliced red bell pepper

$\frac{1}{2}$ cup fresh spinach leaves

8 sun-dried tomatoes, packed in oil, drained and thinly sliced

1. Prepare the noodles according to package directions.

2. While the noodles are cooking, heat the oil in a large skillet over medium heat. Add the garlic and sauté for 1 minute. Add the zucchini, carrots, peas, and red pepper, and sauté for 2 to 3 additional minutes. Add the spinach and tomatoes, and cook just until the spinach wilts.

3. Drain the noodles and transfer to a large bowl. Pour the vegetable mixture over the noodles, toss to coat, and serve.

ROASTED POTATOES

YIELD: 4 SERVINGS

I pound yams, peeled and cut into I-inch cubes

I pound red and white potatoes, scrubbed and diced into I-inch cubes

$\frac{1}{4}$ cup olive oil

I clove garlic, finely chopped

Salt and pepper to taste

I teaspoon dried thyme

I teaspoon dried rosemary

1. Preheat the oven to 400°F.

2. Arrange the potatoes in a large metal baking dish. Drizzle the olive oil over the potatoes and lightly stir until evenly coated. Add the garlic and seasonings, and stir to distribute evenly.

3. Bake uncovered for 45 minutes to an hour, or until tender, stirring the potatoes every 15 minutes. Serve hot.

GREEN LENTILS WITH GARLIC AND CILANTRO

YIELD: 4 SERVINGS

I tablespoon olive oil

I small onion, finely chopped

2 cloves garlic, minced

Two 1-inch pieces fresh ginger, peeled and finely chopped

I teaspoon cumin seeds

$1/4$–$1/2$ cup chopped fresh cilantro

$2 1/2$ cups water

$1 1/3$ cups dried green lentils

I tablespoon fresh lemon juice

Dash red pepper

Salt

1. Place the oil in a large saucepan over medium heat. Add the onion and garlic and cook for about 5 minutes, stirring occasionally, or until the onion is softened and lightly browned.

2. Stir the ginger and cumin into the onion mixture, and cook for 1 minute. Add the cilantro, and stir until it wilts.

3. Add the water and lentils to the pot, and bring to a boil. Reduce the heat, cover, and simmer for 35 to 40 minutes, or until the lentils are tender, adding more water if necessary.

4. Add the lemon juice, red pepper, and salt to the lentils, and simmer for 5 additional minutes, stirring occasionally. Serve hot.

MARINATED BUCKWHEAT SALAD

<u>YIELD: 4 SERVINGS</u>

$^1/_2$ cup buckwheat

1 cup boiling water

$^1/_4$ cup olive oil

2 large cloves garlic, peeled and chopped

3 scallions, chopped

1 large tomato, diced

1 medium lemon, chopped

2 tablespoons coarsely chopped fresh parsley

1 tablespoon coarsely chopped fresh mint

Salt to taste

4 large lettuce leaves

1. Place the buckwheat in a large heatproof mixing bowl. Cover with the boiling water and let stand for 1 hour. Drain.

2. Place the buckwheat in a large bowl, and stir in all of the other ingredients except for the lettuce leaves. Cover and refrigerate for 1 to 2 hours to allow the flavors to blend.

3. Place a lettuce leaf on each of 4 individual serving plates. Spoon a quarter of the buckwheat salad over each leaf, and serve.

Variation

If you cannot find buckwheat or don't like its flavor, try wheat berries, quinoa, or brown rice, and cook the grain according to package directions.

FRESH SALSA

YIELD: ABOUT 3 CUPS

6 medium tomatoes, seeded and chopped

¼ cup fresh lemon juice

I clove garlic

I teaspoon salt

½ onion, minced

½ cup chopped fresh cilantro

I jalapeño pepper, seeded and chopped

1. Place half of the tomatoes, lemon juice, garlic, and salt in a food processor or blender, and process briefly.

2. Transfer the processed tomato mixture to a medium-sized bowl, and stir in all of the remaining ingredients, mixing well. Serve at room temperature or chilled.

PESTO LATINO

YIELD: ABOUT I CUP

2½ cups chopped fresh cilantro

⅔ cup walnuts

⅔ cup fresh lime or lemon juice

½ cup fresh spinach (optional)

I tablespoon minced garlic

I tablespoon minced fresh ginger

I–2 teaspoons minced seeded jalapeño pepper

I½ teaspoons Bragg Liquid Aminos

1. Place all of the ingredients in a food processor or blender, and process into a green cream. Use at room temperature.

CONCLUSION

By the time you have finished the 14-Day Diet, you should be experiencing better health and renewed energy. To maintain these benefits, continue to create meals that are 80 percent alkalizing and 20 percent acidifying, and drink plenty of pure, filtered water and at least one green drink a day. This will help your body to reestablish and then maintain a proper acid-alkaline balance, keeping you on the road to optimal vitality. I predict that once you start to experience the health benefits of this eating plan, you will never want to eat any other way.

Conclusion

I n the Introduction, I told you that I had the answer to our nation's health-care crisis. Now that you have read this book, I hope you can see that we have the power to prevent the misery caused by chronic illness and disease. And we can also slow down and reverse the cost of maintaining our present health-care system—a system that is failing us. But this is the big picture. In order to make this happen, we have to begin with ourselves—one person at a time, one family at a time. The real answer to this crisis is what you can do about your own health, not what others can do when you are sick.

By reading this book, you have provided yourself with the tools you need to effectively rebuild your health. More importantly, you now understand how dependent your health and overall well-being is on a proper acid-alkaline balance, a fact that is entirely overlooked by so many professional health-care practitioners regardless of their specialty and training. This knowledge gives you the ability to take control of your health to a large degree simply with the choices you make each day.

I realize that much of the information provided in this book is new to you, as are my dietary and nutritional recommendations. As a result, you may initially find yourself resisting some of my suggestions. That's normal. But put your skepticism aside and try them out anyway. If you do, I'm confident that it won't be long before you experience better health, improved energy, greater alertness, and greater feelings of well-being.

Even then, however, you may find yourself reverting to old habits from time to time. That's only normal, and if it happens, do not get discouraged. Simply do the best you can, and allow yourself to progress slowly but surely. Change is not easy, even when it is positive, but the more you commit yourself to following the principles discussed throughout this book, the easier it will be to apply them. With a little bit of patience and persistence, it won't be long before you, too, find that your health is in balance for life. While I can't be with you in person, I hope the spirit of this book provides you with the encouragement, information, and direction you need to take the next step.

Glossary of Terms

Acid. Any substance in the body that gives off hydrogen ions when it is dissolved in water. Such substances have a pH value of less than 7.0. *See also* pH.

Acid-alkaline balance. A necessary element of health created by a balanced state of acidic and alkaline substances in the body's fluids and tissues.

Acidifying. Producing an acid state.

Acidosis. A state of chronic over-acidity in the body's tissues and fluids.

Adenosine triphosphate (ATP). A fuel synthesized by the cells from oxygen and glucose. ATP is essential for powering the cells' sodium-potassium pumps, which maintain the proper balance of sodium and potassium within and without the cell walls.

Aerobic. A term literally meaning "with oxygen." This term is used to designate any activity that involves or improves oxygen consumption by the body.

Aerobic exercise. Any form of exercise that enhances the body's utilization of oxygen. Aerobic exercises include jogging, rebounding, running, swimming, and cycling.

Alkaline. Having a pH value greater than 7.0.

Alkalis. Substances that can neutralize acids and that have a pH value greater than 7.0.

Alkalizing. Producing an alkaline state.

Alkalosis. A state of excessive or over-alkalinity in the body's tissues and fluids. Although rare, a state of chronic alkalosis can be life-threatening.

Alternative medicine. A system of medical approaches that do not rely upon drugs and surgery and other conventional Western medical practices. This type of medical care is also known as complementary health care, holistic medicine, and natural healing.

Amino acid. One of the molecular units used by the body to synthesize proteins. Some amino acids are produced by the body, while others must be provided by the diet.

Anaerobic. A term literally meaning "without oxygen." In the human body, an anaerobic state is ideal for the growth of harmful microorganisms such as bacteria, fungi, and viruses.

Aneurysm. An abnormal enlargement of a blood vessel, usually an artery or vein, caused by disease or by weakening of the wall of the vessel.

ANS. *See* Autonomic nervous system.

Antioxidant. Any substance that prevents or slows the process of oxidation, which produces cell-damaging free radicals. Antioxidant nutrients include vitamins A, C, and E; beta-carotene; selenium; and zinc.

Arrhythmia. An abnormal or irregular heartbeat.

Arteriosclerosis. A chronic condition characterized by thickening, loss of elasticity, and hardening of the arteries, resulting in impaired circulation.

ATP. *See* Adenosine triphosphate.

Autonomic nervous system (ANS). The part of the nervous system responsible for controlling and regulating the body's involuntary functions, such as breathing and circulation. The autonomic nervous system consists of two parts: the sympathetic and the parasympathetic nervous systems. *See also* Parasympathetic nervous system; Sympathetic nervous system.

Base. Any substance that reacts with acids to form salts.

Bicarbonate. The most important buffer in the blood. Bicarbonate prevents the blood from becoming too acid or too alkaline.

Biochemical individuality. A term coined by biochemist Roger Williams, PhD, to describe each person's unique genetic makeup and predisposition, unique metabolism, and specific dietary and nutritional needs.

Candida albicans. A yeast that occurs naturally in the gastrointestinal tract and, when overgrown, can create a variety of disease symptoms and lead to candidiasis, or systemic yeast infection.

Candidiasis. A chronic and systemic yeast infection caused by overgrowth of the yeast *Candida albicans.* Also known simply as candida, candidiasis can result in a variety of disease conditions, including allergy, chronic fatigue syndrome, and impaired immunity.

Carcinogen. Any substance, such as an environmental toxin, that can cause cancer.

Carcinogenic. Cancer-causing.

Central nervous system. The main information-processing organs of the nervous system, consisting of the brain and spinal cord.

CFS. *See* Chronic fatigue syndrome.

Chronic fatigue syndrome (CFS). An illness characterized by severe and prolonged exhaustion, often accompanied by depression, headache, mental confusion, mild fever, muscle ache or weakness, and/or sore throat. Because its cause is not a known specific agent, it is referred to as a syndrome rather than a disease.

CMV. *See* Cytomegalovirus.

Coronavirus. A type of virus that is responsible for some, but not all, common colds, and is highly dependent on an acidic environment. It received its name because of its crown-like appearance under a microscope.

Cystitis. Inflammation of the bladder.

Cytomegalovirus (CMV). A common virus of the herpes family. Recent research indicates that the virus is present in the heart tissue of 85 percent of the population and may play an indirect role in heart disease.

Demineralization. A loss of minerals from the body. In a state of chronic acidity, demineralization occurs when the body uses its stores of calcium and other alkalizing minerals to buffer acid wastes.

Diet monotony. The tendency to eat the same foods day in and day out, and thus severely limit the variety of nutrients consumed.

Edema. A condition in which excess fluid accumulates in the body tissues, resulting in swelling of certain body parts, most commonly the feet and legs.

EFAs. *See* Essential fatty acids.

Electrolyte. Any substance which, in a liquid form, is capable of conducting an electric current through the body. Acids, bases, and salts are common forms of electrolytes. Electrolytes help regulate fluid levels in the body, maintain proper pH, and play a vital role in the transmission of nerve impulses from the brain to the rest of the body.

Endocrine system. The body system that produces and regulates the secretion of hormones. The major glands that make up this system include the hypothalamus, pituitary gland, thyroid and parathyroids, adrenal gland, pancreas, testes (in men), and ovaries (in women).

Environmental illness. An illness caused by exposure to pollutants and toxins in the environment—the air, water, and/or land. Such illnesses can include otherwise unexplained allergies, anxiety and depression, arrhythmia, behavioral problems, chronic fatigue syndrome, eczema and hives, edema, gastrointestinal disorders, headache, muscle ache, respiratory conditions, and sleep disorders.

Environmental toxins. Chemicals and other substances released into the environment—the air, water, and/or land—that are hazardous to humans and other animals.

Enzymes. Substances produced by the body and obtained from certain foods—primarily fruits and vegetables—that act as catalysts for biochemical reactions. Enzymes are necessary for every single process that the body performs, including breathing, digestion, immune function, reproduction, and organ function, as well as speech, thought, and movement. A certain class of enzymes, known as digestive enzymes, are available as nutritional supplements to assist in the digestion of carbohydrates, fats, fibers, and proteins.

Essential fatty acids (EFAs). Fats required by the body's cells to ensure proper cell function. Essential fatty acids cannot be manufactured by the body, and therefore must be supplied by the diet in order to ensure good health. There are two primary sources of EFAs: omega-3 fatty acids and omega-6 fatty acids.

Fibromyalgia. A condition characterized by widespread muscle pain, which may be accompanied by anxiety, chronic fatigue, dizziness, headache, numbness or tingling sensations, and/or sleep disorders.

Frankenfoods. A disparaging term coined to describe genetically engineered foods that are not naturally occurring. *See also* Genetically engineered foods.

Free radical. An unstable molecule that attacks other molecules, causing them, too, to become free radicals. Free radicals naturally occur in the body during energy production, but are created in unhealthy amounts when there is a buildup of toxins and waste products in the body, or when diet is poor and results in nutritional deficiencies. When free radical production becomes excessive, cellular damage occurs, leading to disease.

General Adaptation Syndrome. A term coined by pioneering stress researcher Hans Selye, MD, to describe the biochemical response to stress. According to Selye, when stress becomes chronic, the body becomes exhausted.

Genetic predisposition. An increased risk of getting a disease based on hereditary factors passed down from generation to generation through the genes.

Genetically engineered foods. Foods created in a laboratory by altering or modifying their genetic structure. Although the manufacturers of such foods maintain that they are safe, critics point out that the long-term effects of eating such foods are not yet known.

Germ theory of disease. The disease theory popularized by Louis Pasteur, who maintained that diseases are caused by exposure to external bacteria, fungi, or viruses, collectively referred to as germs.

HCl. *See* Hydrochloric acid.

Heat shock protein. A type of protein required by the body to facilitate cellular repair.

Homeostasis. The body's inherent self-regulating mechanisms, which seek always to maintain equilibrium, or balance, within all of the body's systems.

Hormone. A chemical messenger sent from one cell to another to help regulate proper cell and organ function, aid in the body's response to stress, and assist in proper metabolism and energy production.

Hydrochloric acid (HCl). An acid secreted by the stomach to activate the digestive enzymes that break down food into small particles for absorption.

Hydrogen ion. A single unstable proton created when hydrogen molecules are dissolved in water through a process known as dissociation. All acids in the body give off hydrogen ions when they are dissolved in water. pH values are determined by the concentration of hydrogen ions in the substance. The greater the concentration of hydrogen ions, the more acidic it is, while a substance with a lesser concentration is considered neutral or alkaline.

Hyperglycemia. High blood sugar caused by higher-than-normal concentrations of glucose in the bloodstream.

Hyperventilation. Extremely rapid or deep breathing that causes a rapid loss of carbon dioxide during exhalation. When the level of carbon dioxide is reduced, the arteries constrict, causing the brain to experience a shortage of oxygen, and resulting in dizziness and fainting.

Hypoglycemia. Low blood sugar caused by lower-than-normal concentrations of glucose in the bloodstream.

Inflammation. A condition caused by acid buildup and characterized by redness, swelling, pain, and a feeling of heat.

Ion. An atom or group of atoms that bears one or more positive or negative electrical charges due to loss or gain of electrons. When ions lose electrons they become positively charged, and when they gain electrons they become negatively charged.

Jaundice. A disease condition caused by liver dysfunction that results in increased amounts of bile pigments entering and remaining in the bloodstream. Jaundice is characterized by abnormally yellowish coloration of the eyes, skin, and/or urine.

Lactic acid. A waste product produced by the breakdown of glucose by the cells. Lactic acid buildup increases acidity in the body, making it difficult for healthy cells to obtain and efficiently make use of oxygen.

Lymph. A clear yellowish fluid that is part of the lymphatic system. Lymph removes bacteria and certain proteins from the cells, carries away excess fluids and returns them to the bloodstream, transports fat from the small intestine, and assists the body in immune function.

Lymphatic system. An integral part of the immune system, the lymphatic system acts as the body's filtration system, helping to eliminate cellular wastes. The system also plays an important role in the defense mechanisms of the body. When the lymphatic system becomes clogged or congested due to buildup of acid wastes, cell function is diminished, setting the stage for disease.

Metabolism. The biochemical reactions and interactions that take place within the body, resulting in the production of energy and the creation of complex substances that form the material of the tissues and organs.

MHV-A59 coronavirus. A strain of coronavirus that thrives in an acidic pH of 6.0 and can cause various types of colds.

Mind/body medicine. The field of medicine that studies the interrelationships between thoughts, emotions, attitudes, and beliefs and their ability to create health and disease. Common types of mind/body medicine include biofeedback therapy, cognitive therapy, guided imagery and visualization, hypnosis, and meditation.

Mitochondria. The cells' internal energy factories. The mitochondria produce energy using a fuel called adenosine triphosphate, a substance synthesized from oxygen and glucose. The mitochondria also play an essential role in all intracellular enzyme activity.

Mole. The term used to describe the molecular weight of a substance. pH is determined by measuring the concentration of hydrogen ions, which is calculated as moles per liter.

Molecule. The smallest particle into which an element or compound can be divided without losing any of its characteristics. The smallest molecular structures consist of a single atom, while a combination of two or more atoms create molecular chemical compounds.

Murine coronavirus A59. A strain of coronavirus that is particularly resistant to the body's immune defense mechanisms when pH levels are 6.0 or lower.

Nephritis. An acute or chronic inflammation of the kidneys.

Neurofunction. The function of the nervous system.

Neuromuscular. Of or involving both the nerves and the muscles.

Neurotransmitter. A molecule that carries signals between neurons (nerve cells), either fostering the initiation of a nerve impulse or inhibiting such an impulse.

Over-alkalinity. A condition characterized by an excessively high alkaline pH.

Parasympathetic nervous system. The part of the autonomic nervous system responsible for conserving the body's energy supply during times of stress. Physiological effects of the parasympathetic nervous system include constriction of the pupils, slowing of the heartbeat, and overall calming effects.

Pathogen. Any microorganism—such as a bacterium, fungus, or virus—capable of causing disease.

Peripheral nerves. All nerves located outside the central nervous system (the brain and spinal cord). The peripheral nerves relay information from the central nervous system to the muscles and other organs, and from other organs back to the brain.

pH. Literally meaning "potential for hydrogen," the term pH refers to a scale of measurement of the acidity or alkalinity of any substance, including body tissues and fluids. The pH scale runs from 0 to 14, with values of 7.0 considered neutral, values below 7.0 considered acidic, and values above 7.0 considered alkaline.

pH Factor. The underlying factor that determines whether the body is in a state of acid-alkaline balance.

pH strip. A type of tape used to measure the pH of saliva or urine.

Pilates. A type of bodywork exercise named after its developer, Joseph H. Pilates. Initially popular with dancers and other performers, the Pilates method is now popular throughout the fitness world. Exercises are performed on the floor or on specialized equipment, and are intended to help coordinate the mind, body, and breath to develop sleek and functionally strong abdominal muscles, a strong and supple back, and aligned shoulders.

Prostatitis. Inflammation of the prostate gland, usually caused by infection.

Psychosocial stress. Stress caused by relationship difficulties, social isolation, and a lack of social support.

Psychospiritual stress. Stress caused by a crisis of faith or values, questions about one's purpose in life, a lack of meaningful work, or an involvement in day-to-day activities that do not reflect one's core beliefs.

Relaxation response. A term coined by Herbert Benson, MD, of Harvard Medical School, to describe the physiological effects produced when the body enters a calm state as a result of meditation or simply sitting still while focusing on one's breathing.

Rhinovirus. A class of viruses that cause many, but not all, forms of the common cold.

Selective serotonin reuptake inhibitors. A class of prescription antidepressant medications that drive serotonin into the cells of the brain. The most widely known drug in this class is Prozac.

Serotonin. A hormone that acts as a "feel good" neurotransmitter in the brain, and influences sleep, mood, and brain functions related to sensory perception.

Sodium-potassium pumps. The mechanisms inside each cell that maintain the proper balance between sodium and potassium within and without the cell walls.

Stressor. An internal or external factor that can trigger stress. Internal stressors include harmful or inaccurate thoughts and beliefs, and suppressed and inappropriately expressed emotions. External stressors include unhealthy foods, environmental toxins, and pathogens.

Subluxation. A misalignment of the spinal vertebrae.

Sympathetic nervous system. The portion of the autonomic nervous system that governs how the body expends energy during times of stress. Physiological effects of the sympathetic nervous system include accelerated heartbeat, increased blood pressure, and dilation of the pupils.

Tai chi. A form of exercise developed in China over two thousand years ago, and characterized by slow stretching movements accompanied by focused breathing and meditative concentration.

Tetany. A disorder characterized by periodic painful muscle spasms and tremors.

Uremia. A condition caused by a buildup of waste products in the blood due to kidney dysfunction. Symptoms include nausea, vomiting, loss of appetite, weakness, and mental confusion.

Venous Plasma pH Test. The most accurate test for measuring the pH of the blood. It needs to be administered by a physician, who withdraws a vial of blood from a vein in the arm, and sends the blood to a licensed laboratory for testing.

Vertebrae. The bone segments that make up the spinal column.

Yeast infection. An infection of the skin or tissue linings caused by fungi. The most common type of yeast infection is candidiasis, caused by overgrowth of the yeast *Candida albicans*.

Yo-yo effect. The rapid weight loss and weight gain that often results from dieting.

Bibliography

Aihara, Herman. *Acid and Alkaline*. Oroville, CA: George Ohsawa Macrobiotic Foundation, 1986.

Appleton, Nancy. *Stopping Inflammation*. Garden City Park, NY: Square One Publishers, 2005.

Brown, Susan E. *Better Bones, Better Body*. Second Edition. Los Angeles: Keats Publishing, 2000.

Gamble, James L., Jr. *Acid-Base Physiology: A Direct Approach*. Baltimore: The Johns Hopkins University Press, 1982.

Guyton, Arthur C., and John E. Hall. *Textbook of Medical Physiology*. Ninth Edition. Philadelphia: W.B. Sanders Company, 1996.

Ivker, Robert; Robert Anderson; and Larry Trivieri, Jr. *The Complete Self-Care Guide to Holistic Medicine*. New York: Tarcher/Putnam, 1999.

Lee, Lita. *The Enzyme Cure*. Tiburon, CA: Future Medicine Publishing, Inc., 1998.

Trivieri, Larry, Jr. *The American Holistic Medical Association Guide to Holistic Health*. New York: John Wiley and Sons, 2001.

Trivieri, Larry, Jr., and John Anderson, Editors. *Alternative Medicine: The Definitive Guide*. Second Edition. Berkeley, CA: Ten Speed/Celestial Arts, 2002.

Vasey, Christopher. *The Acid-Alkaline Diet*. Rochester, VT: Healing Arts Press, 1999.

Index

A

Acid reflux, 70
Acid-alkaline balance of body, importance of, 13–16
Acidifying foods, 80–85
  food charts of, 92–99
Acidosis
  and accelerated aging, 48–49, 72–73
  and allergies, 63–64
  and anxiety, 63–64
  and arthritis, 64–65
  and brain function, 49
  and cancer, 66–67
  and cardiovascular disease, 67
  and cell function, 59–61
  and demineralization, 47, 49–50
  and depression, 63–64
  and diabetes, 68
  and fatigue, 50–51, 68–69
  and gastrointestinal disorders, 70
  and gout, 65–66
  and growth of harmful microorganisms, 53
  and immune function, 52
  and impaired enzyme activity, 51–52
  and inflammation, 52
  and kidney disease, 70–71
  and obesity, 75–76
  and osteoporosis, 71–72
  and respiratory conditions, 73–74
  and skin problems, 52, 74
  and vision problems, 74–74
  and weight gain, 75–76
Acids
  body's elimination of, 42–44
  body's neutralization of, 45–47
Adenosine triphosphate (ATP), 69
Aging, accelerated, 48–49, 72–73
Air, improving, 32–33
Alcohol, dangers of, 23, 25, 81
  avoiding, on 14-Day Diet, 128–129
Alkalizing food, 86–91
  food charts of, 92–99
Alkalosis
  causes of, 47
  side effects of, 48
Allergies, 63
Almonds, 83

*Alternative Medicine Definitive
Guide to Cancer, An*
(Diamond and Cowden), 66
*American Holistic Medical
Association Guide to Holistic
Health, The* (Trivieri), 12
Amylase, 118–119
Anaerobic environments,
dangers of, 50–51. *See also*
Cancer.
Anderson, Robert A., 5, 9, 81, 84,
103
Aneurysm, 67
Anxiety, 63–64
Arrhythmia, 67
Arteriosclerosis, 67
Arthritis, 64–65
Artificial sweeteners, as
acidifying foods, 85
Ascorbic acid (vitamin C),
108–109
Asthma, 5
ATP. *See* Adenosine
triphosphate.
Attention deficit hyperactivity
disorder (ADHD), 5
Attitudes and beliefs,
importance of improving,
36–37
Autism, 5
Autonomic nervous system
(ANS), 11

B

Bacteria, proliferation of
harmful, 53
Batmanghelidj, F., 9, 26
Beans. *See* Legumes.
Beliefs and attitudes, importance
of improving, 36–37

Benson, Herbert, 35
Beta-carotene, 107
Better Bones, Better Body (Brown),
50, 71
Beverages, chart of, 98
Blackened Tofu, 151
Bladder stones, 71
Blood pH, 41
determining, 54–55
Boron, 111
Brain pH, 41
Brazil nuts, 83
Bread
as acidifying food, 81, 94
avoiding, on 14-Day Diet, 128
Breakfast Burrito, 142
Breakfast Olé, 140
Breathing, role of, in eliminating
acids, 44
Breathing exercises
to promote relaxation, 34–35
to promote sleep, 31
Broccoli Ziti with Garlic, 155
Brown, Susan E., 50, 71–72, 112
Buckwheat Salad, Marinated, 158
Burrito, Breakfast, 142

C

Caffeine, dangers of, 23
Caffeine products, as acidifying
foods, 81
Calcium, 111–112
Cancer, 66–67
Candidiasis, spread of, due to
acid-alkaline imbalance, 15
Cardiovascular disease, 67
Cataracts, 75
Cell function, disruption of, due
to acid-alkaline imbalance,
14, 59–60

Cellulase, 119
CFS. *See* Chronic fatigue
 syndrome.
Chamomile tea, benefits of, 30
Cheese. *See* Dairy products.
Chemicals, toxic, use of, 12–13
Chicken, Garlic, 150
Chicken Salad, 147
Children and obesity, 5
Chili, Veggie, 145
Chlorophyll, benefits of, 90
 in green drinks, 122
Chronic fatigue syndrome
 (CFS), 6, 51. *See also* Fatigue.
Cleansing diet. *See* 14-Day Diet.
Coffee, avoiding, on 14-Day
 Diet, 129
Cold, common, 73
Colitis, 70
Commercial farming methods,
 7, 24
Commercial meat industry, 7–8
*Complete Self-Care Guide to
 Holistic Medicine, The* (Ivker
 and Anderson), 5, 84
Condiments
 as acidifying foods, 81–82, 99
 avoiding, on 14-Day Diet, 129
Conscious breathing, 35. *See also*
 Breathing exercises.
Constipation, 70
Copper, 112–113
Coronavirus, 73
Cowden, W. Lee, 66
Crohn's disease, 70
Curried Chicken Salad, 148–149

D

Dairy products
 as acidifying foods, 83, 94

avoiding, on 14-Day Diet, 129
Dehydration, chronic, 9
Demineralization, 47, 49–50
Depression, 63–64
Determining your pH, 54–58
Diabetes, 68
Diamond, W. John, 66
Diarrhea, 70
Diet
 as cornerstone of good
  health, 20–21
 14-Day. *See* 14-Day Diet.
 guidelines for, 21–23, 78–79
 standard American. *See*
  Standard American diet.
 See also Foods.
Diet monotony, 8
Digestive enzymes. *See* Enzyme
 supplements.
Disaccharidase, 119–120.
Diverticulitis, 70
Dried fruits, 86–87, 97
Drugs. *See* Medications.
Dyslexia, 5
Dyspepsia, 70

E

Eating habits, unhealthy
 American. *See* Standard
 American diet.
Eczema, 74
Edison, Thomas, 18
EFAs. *See* Essential fatty acids.
Eggplant and Tofu, Roasted, 153
Electrolytes, balance of, 51
Environmental illness, 6
Enzyme activity, impaired,
 51–52, 69
Enzyme deficiencies, 118
Enzyme Nutrition (Howell), 51

Enzyme supplements, 52, 117
    amylase, 118–119
    cellulase, 119
    disaccharidase, 119–120
    lipase, 120
    protease, 120
Essential fatty acids (EFAs)
    food sources of, 117
    importance of, 21, 116–117
    supplements of, 117
Exercise, importance of, 9–10,
    27–29
    programs, recommended, 28
    specific benefits of, 27–28, 31

F

Farming. *See* Commercial
    farming methods.
Fast food, dangers of, 22
Fatigue, 50–51, 68–69. *See also*
    Chronic fatigue syndrome.
Fats and oils, chart of, 98–99
Fiber, importance of, 22
Fibromyalgia, 6
Fiesta Toast, 144
Fish, as acidifying food, 82, 95
Flatulence, 70
Florentine-Stuffed Tomatoes, 152
Folacin (folic acid), 109–110
Folate (folic acid), 109–110
Food charts, 92–99
Food quality, poor, 7–8
Foods
    acidifying, 80–85
    alkalizing, 86–91
    charts of alkalizing and
        acidifying foods, 92–99
    effect of, on pH levels, 77–78
    guidelines for choosing,
        21–23, 78–79

tips for combining, 99–101
14-Day Diet
    basic guidelines for, 125–128
    foods to avoid during,
        128–129
    nonvegetarian menus for,
        130–135
    recipes for, 140–159
    vegetarian menus for,
        135–139
Fresh Salsa, 159
Fruit juices, avoiding, on
    14-Day Diet, 129
Fruits
    as acidifying foods, 86, 96–97
    as alkalizing foods, 86–87,
        96-97
    avoiding, on 14-Day Diet,
        125–126
    dried, 86–87, 97
    importance of, 21
    when to eat, 100
Fungi, proliferation of harmful,
    53

G

Garlic Chicken, 150
Gastrointestinal disorders, 70
General Adaptation Syndrome,
    11–12
Genetically altered foods, 8
Genetically modified organism
    (GMO), 8
GMO. See Genetically modified
    organism, 8
Gout, 65–66
Grains, as acidifying foods, 82, 93
Green drinks, 121–123
    guidelines for making and
        using, 124, 130

Green Lentils with Garlic and Cilantro, 157
Guyton, Arthur C., 14, 41, 47, 48

H

Hay, William Howard, 13
Health-care costs, rising, 6
Healthy Pleasures (Ornstein and Sobel), 37
Heart attack, 67
Heart pH, 41
Heartburn, 46
Heat shock protein, 49
Herbal teas, benefits of, 30
Herbs and spices, as alkalizing foods, 87, 99
Hippocrates, 20, 77
Home and work environments, healthy, 32–33
Hops tea, benefits of, 30
"How Healthy Are You?" Quiz, 19
Howell, Edward, 51
Humidifiers, 33
Humor, cultivating, 37
Hydrochloric acid (HCl)
    and heartburn, 46
    and over-acidity, 46
    role of, in digestion, 45–46
Hydrogen ions and pH, 40
Hypertension, 67

I

Indigestion, 70
Irradiation, 8
Irritable bowel syndrome (IBS), 70
Italian Soup, 144–145
Ivker, Robert S., 5, 9, 33, 81, 84, 103

J

Junk food, dangers of, 22

K

Kidney disease, 70–71
Kidney stones, 71
Kidneys, role of, in eliminating acids, 42, 44
Koop, C. Everett, 6

L

Labels on nutritional supplements, understanding, 105–106
Laughter, benefits of, 37
Learned Optimism (Seligman), 36
Leftovers, avoiding, on 14-Day Diet, 129
Legumes as acidifying foods, 82–83, 95
Lentils with Garlic and Cilantro, Green, 157
Lipase, 120
Lipton, Bruce, 10
Liver pH, 41

M

Macular degeneration, 75
Magnesium, 113
Maimonides, 20
Marinated Buckwheat Salad, 158
Meat, as acidifying food, 82, 95
Meat industry. *See* Commercial meat industry.
Medications, acid-producing nature of, 61–62
Meditation, benefits of, 35
Mediterranean Moussaka, 154–155

Methyl sulfonyl methane
   (MSM). See MSM.
MHV-A59 coronavirus, 73
Microorganisms, growth of
   harmful, 53–54
Milk. See Dairy products.
Minerals
   lack of, in soil, 7, 24
   loss of, due to over-acidity,
      47, 49–50
Minerals, essential, 110
   boron, 111
   calcium, 111–112
   copper, 112–113
   magnesium, 113
   phosphorus, 113–114
   potassium, 114–115
   silica, 115
   zinc, 115–116
Molds, proliferation of harmful, 53
Molecule, definition of, 40
Moussaka, Mediterranean,
   154–155
MSM (methyl sulfonyl
   methane), 120–121
Muffins, Oat Bran, 141
Murine coronavirus A59, 73
Muscle pH, 41
Muscle tension, soothing, 34

N

Negative ion generators, 33
Nephritis, 70
New Health Era, A (Hay), 13
Nutritional supplements. See
   Supplements, nutritional.
Nuts
   as acidifying foods, 83–84, 96
   as alkalizing foods, 87, 96
   avoiding, on 14-Day Diet, 129

O

Oat Bran Muffins, 141
Obesity
   and acidosis, 75–76
   American epidemic of, 5, 7
   health problems caused by, 7
Oils, cold-pressed, as alkalizing
   foods, 87, 99
Oils and fats, chart of, 98–99
Omega-3 fats, 21
Omega-6 fats, 21
Omelet, Vegetable, 140–141
Orange Roughy with Butter
   Sauce and Almonds, 149
Organic foods, importance of, 21
Ornstein, Robert, 37
Osteoarthritis, 64–65
Osteoporosis, 50, 71–72
Over-acidity, chronic, 41
   body's attempts to cope with,
      44
   loss of minerals due to, 47
   See also Acidosis; Acids.

P

Parasympathetic nervous
   system, 11–12
Pasta Primavera, 156
Pathogens, susceptibility to,
   due to acid-alkaline
   imbalance, 15
Pesticides, use of, 12
Pesto Latino, 159
pH
   of blood, 14, 41
   body's regulation of, 42–47
   and cell health, 59–61
   determining, 54–58
   imbalances, harmful effects
      of, 47–54, 63–76

understanding values of,
39–40

values, of the human body, 41

See also Acidosis; Alkalosis.

pH eating plans, 78–80

pH strips, use of, 55–58

Phosphorus, 113–114

Physical stress, 11

Pollution, health risks of, 12

Potassium, 114–115

Potatoes, as alkalizing food, 91

Potatoes, Roasted, 156–157

Poultry, as acidifying food, 82, 95

Processed foods, as acidifying, 83

Processed meats, avoiding, on
14-Day Diet, 129

Protease, 120

Psoriasis, 74

Psychological stress, 11

Psychosocial stress, 11

Psychospiritual stress, 11

Pyridoxine (Vitamin B_6), 107–108

Q

Quiz, "How Healthy Are You?,"
19

R

Recipes for 14-Day Diet, 140–159

Red Lettuce and Radish Sprout
Salad, 148

Refined carbohydrates, dangers
of, 23

Relaxation. *See* Relaxation
exercises; Sleep and
relaxation; Stress.

Relaxation exercises, 34–35

Relaxation response, 35

Respiratory conditions, 73–74

Rheumatoid arthritis, 65

Roasted Eggplant and Tofu, 153

Roasted Potatoes, 156–157

S

Salads
Chicken, 147
Curried Chicken, 148–149
Marinated Buckwheat, 158
Red Lettuce and Radish
Sprout, 148
Spinach and Egg, 146

Saliva pH, 41

Salsa, Fresh, 159

Salt, dangers of, 23

Salt, sea and Celtic, as alkalizing
food, 87, 99

Saturated fats, dangers of, 22–23

Sedentary lifestyle, health risks
of, 9–10

Seeds, as acidifying foods,
83–84, 96

Selective serotonin reuptake
inhibitors (SSRIs), 64

Seligman, Martin, 36

Selye, Hans, 11

Sense of humor, cultivating, 37

Serotonin levels, 63–64

Silica, 115

Silicon (silica), 115

Sinus Survival (Ivker), 33

Skin conditions, 74

Skin pH, 41

Sleep and relaxation
importance of, 30
ways of promoting, 30–32,
33–37

Smoked meats, avoiding, on
14-Day Diet, 129

Snacks, choosing, for 14-Day
Diet, 127

Sobel, David, 37
Soda, as acidifying food, 84, 98
Sodium, influence of, on health, 42–43
Soil, poor mineral content of, 7, 24
Sorensen, Soren Peter Lauritz, 39
Soup, Italian, 144–145
Soup, Vegetable, 143
Spinach and Egg Salad, 146
Spine health, importance of, 29
Sprouts
    as alkalizing food, 88
    growing, 89
SSRIs. *See* Selective serotonin reuptake inhibitors.
Standard American diet, as cause of death and illness, 5–7
Stomach problems, 70
Stress
    gaining relief from, 31, 33–37
    health risks of, 10–12
Subluxation, 29
Sugar
    as acidifying food, 84–85
    avoiding, on 14-Day Diet, 128
    dangers of, 22
Supplements, nutritional
    digestive enzymes, 117–120
    essential fatty acids, 116–117
    green drinks, 121–123
    guidelines for choosing, 104–106
    guidelines for using, 123, 124
    labels, reading, 105–106
    mineral, 110–116
    MSM, 120–121
    need for, 24, 103–104
    suggested, 104–123
    vitamin, 107–110

Sweat glands, role of, in eliminating acids, 44
Sympathetic nervous system, 11

T

Tea, avoiding, on 14-Day Diet, 129
Teenagers and obesity, 5
Test, "How Healthy Are You?," 19
Tetany, 48
Textbook of Medical Physiology, The (Guyton), 14, 41
Toast, Fiesta, 144
Tofu, Blackened, 151
Tofu, Roasted Eggplant and, 153
Tomatoes, Florentine-Stuffed, 152
Tooth problems, 50
Toxins, environmental, proliferation of, 12–13
Transcendental Meditation, 35
Trans-fatty acids, dangers of, 22
Trivieri, Larry, Jr., 12
Tuna-Stuffed Avocado, 147
Type II diabetes, 68

U

Uremia, 71
Uric acid, 65
Urine, changes in color and odor of, 45
Urine pH, 41
    determining, 55–58

V

Valerian root tea, benefits of, 31
Variety in diet, importance of, 21. *See also* Diet monotony.
Vegetable Omelet, 140–141
Vegetable Soup, 143

Vegetables, importance of, 21
     as alkalizing foods, 88, 92–93
Veggie Chili, 145
Venous plasma pH test, 54–55
Vinegar, avoiding, on 14-Day
     Diet, 129
Viruses, proliferation of, 53
Vision problems, 74–75
Vitamins, essential
     A, 107
     B$_6$, 107–108
     B$_{12}$, 108
     C, 108–109
     D, 109
     folic acid, 109–110

W

Warburg, Otto, 66
Water
     as alkalizing food, 86
     body's need for, 9, 25–26
     dangers of inadequate intake
          of, 25–26
     guidelines for healthy intake
          of, 26–27
     need for pure, 27
     tap, as acidifying, 85
     when to drink, 100
Water and lemon juice,
          guidelines for making, 130
Weight gain, 75–76. *See also*
     Obesity.
We're Eating Ourselves to Death, 5
West, Samuel, 69

Y

Yeast products, as acidifying
     foods, 85
     avoiding, on 14-Day Diet, 128
Yeasts, proliferation of harmful,
     53
Your Body's Many Cries for Water
     (Batmanghelidj), 9, 26

Z

Zinc, 115–116
Ziti with Garlic, Broccoli, 155

RELIEVING PAIN NATURALLY
Safe and Effective Alternative Approaches
To Treating and Overcoming Chronic Illness

Sylvia Goldfarb, PhD
and Robrta W. Waddell

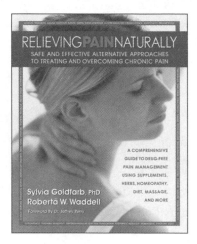

For millions of Americans, severe pain is a fact of everyday life. Standard medicine commonly offers relief through drug therapies. While often effective, these medications come with a host of side effects— disorientation, drowsiness, mental impairment, nausea, peptic ulcers, tinnitus, and addiction, to mention just a few. Moreover, after prolonged use, the body's tolerance to many of these drugs requires increased dosages to remain effective. While many sufferers would prefer nondrug options, much of the available information on alternative pain treatment is scattered, incomplete, self-serving, and in many instances, out of date—or it was, until now. Professional health writers Dr. Sylvia Goldfarb and Roberta Waddell have designed *Relieving Pain Naturally* to be a comprehensive guide to drug-free pain management. Here is an up-to-date resource that is written in clear nontechnical language for ease of use and quick accessibility.

Relieving Pain Naturally is divided into two parts. Part One examines over forty of the most common chronic pain-related conditions, from abdominal pain to sciatica to tendonitis. Each disorder is explained, and its alternative pain treatments detailed. Part Two offers twenty-seven drug-free therapies. These entries include both conventional treatments and alternative modalities such as acupuncture, biofeedback, heat and cold therapy, hypnosis, nutrition, and oxygen therapy. Also included are clinical studies and cautions, where applicable. A comprehensive resource guide provides a list of groups and professional organizations that can help you find the appropriate therapist in your area.

For years, millions of pain sufferers have longed for a safe, side effect-free treatment for chronic pain, but have been unsure how to take that first step towards greater health. Now, *Relieving Pain Naturally* provides a reliable starting point.

$18.95 • 296 pages • 8.5 x 11-inch Quality trade paperback • Health • ISBN 0-7570-0079-7

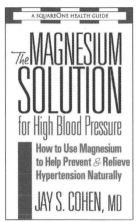

THE MAGNESIUM SOLUTION FOR HIGH BLOOD PRESSURE
How to Use Magnesium to Help Prevent and Relieve Hypertension Naturally
Jay S. Cohen, MD

Approximately 50 percent of all Americans have hypertension, a devastating disease that can lead to hardening of the arteries, heart attack, and stroke. While many medications are available to combat this condition, these drugs come with potentially dangerous side effects. When Dr. Jay S. Cohen learned of his own vascular condition, he was well aware of the risks associated with standard treatments. Based upon his research, he selected a safer option—magnesium.

In *The Magnesium Solution for High Blood Pressure,* Dr. Cohen describes the most effective types of magnesium for treating hypertension, explores appropriate magnesium dosage, and details the use of magnesium in conjunction with hypertension meds. Here is a proven remedy for anyone looking for a safe, effective approach to the treatment of high blood pressure.

$5.95 • 96 pages • 4 x 7.5-inch mass paperback • Health/High Blood Pressure • ISBN 0-7570-0255-2

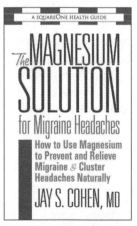

THE MAGNESIUM SOLUTION FOR MIGRAINE HEADACHES
How to Use Magnesium to Prevent and Relieve Migraine and Cluster Headaches Naturally
Jay S. Cohen, MD

More than 30 million people across North America suffer from migraine headaches. Over the years, a number of drugs have been developed to treat migraines, but these treatments don't work for everyone, and come with a high risk of side effects. Fortunately, Dr. Jay S. Cohen has discovered an alternative—magnesium.

This easy-to-understand guide explains what a migraine is, and shows how magnesium can play a key role in preventing and treating migraine headaches. It also describes what type of magnesium works best, and how much magnesium should be taken to prevent or stop migraines. For those who are looking for a safe and effective approach to the prevention and treatment of migraine and cluster headaches, Dr. Cohen prescribes a proven natural remedy in *The Magnesium Solution for Migraine Headaches.*

$5.95 • 96 pages • 4 x 7.5-inch mass paperback • Health/Migraines • ISBN 0-7570-0256-0

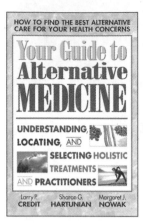

YOUR GUIDE TO ALTERNATIVE MEDICINE

Understanding, Locating, and Selecting Holistic Treatments and Practitioners

Larry P. Credit, Sharon G. Hartunian, and Margaret J. Nowak

The growing world of complementary medicine offers safe and effective solutions to many health disorders, from allergies to backaches to headaches. You may already be interested in alternative care approaches, but if you're like most people, you have a hundred and one questions you'd like answered before you choose a treatment. "Will I feel the acupuncture needles?" "Does chiropractic hurt?" "What is a homeopathic remedy?" "Does massage really work?" The fact is that the more you know about these alternative health-care techniques, the greater your chance of selecting the right remedy for your own health problem. *Your Guide to Alternative Medicine* provides the fundamental facts necessary to choose an effective complementary care therapy and begin treatment.

This comprehensive reference clearly explains numerous approaches in an easy-to-read format. For every complementary care option discussed, there is a description and brief history; a list of conditions that respond; an explanation of how the therapy works; information on the cost and duration of treatment; a discussion of what you should expect regarding the credentials and educational background of practitioners; a directory of professional organizations that can offer you further information; recommended readings; and more. To find those therapies most appropriate for a specific condition, there is even a unique troubleshooting chart that lists common disorders along with the complementary approaches best suited to treat them.

Your Guide to Alternative Medicine introduces you to options that you may never have considered—techniques that enhance the body's natural healing potential and have few, if any, side effects. Here is a reference that can help you make informed decisions about all your important health-care needs.

---

*$11.95 • 208 pages • 6 x 9-inch quality paperback • Health/Alternative Therapies/Reference
ISBN 0-7570-0125-4*